TACKLING POVERTY AND SOCIAL EXCLUSION

In our highly unequal Britain poverty and social exclusion continue to dominate the lives of users of social work and social care services. At the same time, spending cuts and welfare reform have changed the context within which services are delivered. The third edition of this unique textbook seeks to capture the complexity and diversity of practice relating to social exclusion as social workers adapt to this challenging environment.

Tackling Poverty and Social Exclusion prepares practitioners to engage directly with the social and personal circumstances facing excluded individuals and their families. The volume:

- explains the development of the concept of social exclusion as a framework for understanding the impact of poverty and other deprivations on users' lives, and outlines five building blocks for combating exclusion in practice;
- locates practice within social work values of fairness and social justice while acknowledging the many challenges to those values;
- includes individual chapters on excluded children and families, young people and adults – with chapters also on practice in disadvantaged neighbourhoods and rural communities; and
- discusses inclusionary practice in relation to racism as well as refugees and asylum seekers.

Throughout, the book encourages students and practitioners to think through the range of approaches, perspectives and value choices they face. To facilitate engagement each chapter includes up-to-date practice examples, case studies and specific questions for readers to reflect on.

John H. Pierson has taught at Staffordshire University for twenty years and is currently Visiting Lecturer in the Creative Communities Unit at Staffordshire University, UK. He is the author of *Understanding Social Work: History and Context* and has co-edited the *Dictionary of Social Work*, among other works.

'In a thought-provoking book, Pierson convincingly argues that social exclusion remains the sometimes ambivalent construct which connects the great majority of welfare service users who come to the attention of social services. Through intelligent case studies, astute theory and meticulous evidence Pierson highlights that social workers need to think hard about the impact which elevated levels of poverty, gross inequality and stigma have upon the too often constrained life chances of many people who turn to an increasingly fragmented social services. This book is a must-read for all students hoping against great odds to meaningfully support people within the seemingly post–Welfare State'.

Professor Malcolm Carey, Head of Social Work, University of Chester, UK

'An excellent guide to social work practice and analysis: for students, educators and practitioners. It highlights the impact of poverty and forms of social exclusion on service users' lives. It takes account of the harsh current context of social work. It shows, nevertheless, how social work that addresses inequality and engages cooperatively with service users, can contribute to fairer shares of social and material resources. Throughout, a realistic grasp of practice informs helpful case studies and exercises'.

Eileen McLeod, Emeritus Associate Professor, University of Warwick, UK

TACKLING POVERTY AND SOCIAL EXCLUSION

Promoting social justice in social work

THIRD EDITION

John H. Pierson

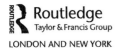
Routledge
Taylor & Francis Group

LONDON AND NEW YORK

First published 2001
Second edition published 2010
by Routledge

This edition published 2016
by Routledge
2 Park Square, Milton Park, Abingdon, Oxon OX14 4RN

and by Routledge
711 Third Avenue, New York, NY 10017

Routledge is an imprint of the Taylor & Francis Group, an informa business

British Library Cataloguing in Publication Data
A catalogue record for this book is available from the British Library

Library of Congress Cataloging-in-Publication Data
Names: Pierson, John, 1944– author.
Title: Tackling poverty and social exclusion : promoting
social justice in social work / John Pierson.
Other titles: Tackling social exclusion
Description: Abingdon, Oxon ; New York, NY : Routledge, 2016. |
Earlier editions published as: Tackling social exclusion.
Identifiers: LCCN 2015041199| ISBN 9780415742986 (hardback) |
ISBN 9780415742993 (pbk.) | ISBN 9781315813967 (ebook)
Subjects: LCSH: Social service. | Marginality, Social. |
Poor. | Social justice.
Classification: LCC HV40 .P535 2016 | DDC 361—dc23
LC record available at http://lccn.loc.gov/2015041199

ISBN: 978-0-415-74298-6 (hbk)
ISBN: 978-0-415-74299-3 (pbk)
ISBN: 978-1-315-81396-7 (ebk)

Typeset in Sabon
by Keystroke, Station Road, Codsall, Wolverhampton

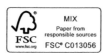
MIX
Paper from
responsible sources
FSC
www.fsc.org   FSC® C013056

Printed and bound in Great Britain by
TJ International Ltd, Padstow, Cornwall

For Frank and Kaz, with love

Without dignity our lives are only blinks of duration. But if we manage to lead a good life well, we create something more. We write a subscript to our mortality. We make our lives tiny diamonds in the cosmic sands.

Ronald Dworkin, Justice for Hedgehogs

CONTENTS

FIGURES AND TABLES

FIGURES

TABLE

ACKNOWLEDGEMENTS

I would like to thank Keith Puttick at Staffordshire University and Martin Thomas at Manchester University for reading portions of this volume as it was being prepared. They alerted me to needed changes.

I would like to thank Craig Cawthorne and John Webb for calling my attention to the work of Brightlife, a partnership for and with older people in Cheshire.

The book benefited from a paper by Adrian Randall on destitution among asylum seekers; I have tried to convey some of his passion and factual analysis of what happens to asylum seekers on the streets of Britain.

Families learning together is a vital approach to tackling exclusion. On this important subject Keith McDowell, head of the Knowsley Family Learning Service, provided me with material on the work that his team undertakes in disadvantaged areas of Liverpool. He and his colleagues deserve immense credit for their achievements.

I owe thanks to my longstanding collaborators and friends Terry Philpot, Simon Ward and Bob Maclaren for our running conversations on politics, social policy and machinations inside universities. To these I add the name of the late Paul Boylan who, over the course of the dozen years as my colleague and friend, proved to be a fount of fresh and committed approaches to work with children and adolescents.

I would like to thank the team at the Malpas Youth Centre: Eric Beak, Sally Sharp, Penny Davies, Steven Schrimshaw and Margo Webb, for our years together working with young people and our discussions of adolescent behaviour along the way.

The librarians at the community library at the Bishop Heber High School secured a wide range of publications from near and far for me. Would that everyone would be so lucky to have a library like this on their doorstep.

Finally I thank Miriam Sharp Pierson for producing the graphics in the volume.

It goes without saying that errors or misstatements are my responsibility.

INTRODUCTION

The first edition of this volume was published in 2001. At that time the concept of social exclusion was fresh and central to government policy as it strove to solve persistent social problems such as young teenage pregnancy, homelessness, long-term adult unemployment and neighbourhood disadvantage. University and think-tank research debated and broadened the concept by tracking the extent of exclusion across the country. Definitions of exclusion were formulated and indicators developed. Heavyweight academic departments such as the Centre for the Analysis of Social Exclusion at the London School of Economics and other independent organisations such as the New Policy Institute amassed evidence, monitored the incidence of exclusion and analysed the processes through which exclusion occurs.

The climate is now vastly different, as readers of this third edition will know. While the Social Exclusion Unit had already been wound up before Labour was voted out of office in 2010 – turning over its work to a Social Exclusion Task Force which itself was then dissolved – the Coalition government elected in 2010 and the subsequent Conservative government of 2015 abandoned the term social exclusion, replacing it with a more nebulous discourse around 'the most vulnerable in our society'.

This does not mean that the phenomenon of exclusion – marginalisation, poverty, powerlessness and isolation – has disappeared in Britain. In fact the opposite has happened, as this volume will comprehensively demonstrate. One of the central arguments of this book is that the impact of the economic recession from 2008 to early 2010, combined with Coalition and Conservative government austerity policies, has created an exclusionary process of unusual depth delivering waves of hardship, inequality and powerlessness across the populations of the United Kingdom.

Within this context a major reorientation of welfare policy has taken place that directly affects social work. The welfare state originally was intended to provide some protection from the labour market to those who needed it – whether the unemployed, the disabled, the long-term sick, those with mental health problems or, of course, children and young people. That mission is now badly frayed. Britain is a country where food banks have assumed a prominent place in the lives of hundreds of thousands of people. Students graduate with unprecedented debt. Public services have been fragmented, privatised and stripped of funding. At its most extreme, in the case of youth services for example, the service has completely disappeared. Those with disability face compulsory testing to prove they can work. Welfare benefits are withdrawn as 'sanctions' from tens of thousands of claimants. Many jobs vital to the economy as a whole and on which even the better-off depend to function well – transport, street cleaning, environmental services, hotel servicing, restaurants, child care, residential care for older people – remain trapped in a low skill and low pay structure.

SOCIAL WORK AND SOCIAL EXCLUSION

Social workers work every day with the socially excluded and in the main the poorest in society. Not only do they help users resolve problems of living but they are also the close-up witness to the deprivation and inequality all around them – of people shorn of defences, resources, skills, hope, self-respect, dignity. This volume aims to build on this role that social workers occupy as both support and witness to those who are at greatest disadvantage. It urges social workers to think hard about inequalities and poverty in our society and what they can do about it.

Social exclusion is the thread that links the great majority of social work service users. It is not a concept to use lightly. It means what it says: *excluded from society* – cut off, denied, without access, marginalised in relation to income, education, parental resources, social networks, job-providing networks. The human dimension of users is not defined by their exclusion, but it is the central circumstance that they have to deal with, and any 'problem-based social work', any professional aspiration to work 'in partnership', any 'full assessment', or anti-oppressive practice that ignores this is incomplete. Work with transgender youth is a good example of how a focus on exclusion broadens, not narrows, social work commitments.

This is why it is important to understand the broader terrain of exclusion. One of the objectives of the volume is to provide a briefing on policy – its direction of travel and implications for practice. Without knowledge of policy and the way it affects people, 'practice' becomes cut off from those forces that are constantly working to reshape it. Allied with this is the second objective: to provide evidence that suggests more effective lines of practice. Practice is not a free-standing realm of techniques and approaches – it only appears that way to practitioners if they have little knowledge of the social environment within which users carry out their lives, or of the evidence drawn from research in the field. Practice is what social workers deliver – what they do when they engage with people – and good practice is what good social workers do, and that includes working for just outcomes in the circumstances that individuals and their families face. What social workers can do about exclusion, what evidence they need to have and what knowledge and value sets they are to draw on is the subject of this volume.

Nevertheless the terrain of social exclusion as in social work practice is made up of differing sets of evidence, competing interpretations that practitioners have to think through. It is imperative for example that social workers understand exactly what those advocating a greater role for markets in service delivery are saying, if for no other reason than that is where so much of policy is headed. Such awareness is crucial whether one is trying to limit marketisation of services or promote it. The principle of different perspectives applies also to the examples and suggestions of practice that appear throughout the volume. These have been drawn from across the country – and when appropriate, from the US and continental Europe – and from the many kinds of social work organisations that are now in the field.

ROAD MAP FOR THE REST OF THE VOLUME

Chapter 1 discusses the elements that make up social exclusion and shows how the concept fits in with other definitions of poverty. Chapter 2 examines the contentious world of values and asks social workers to think through their individual values, particularly in relation to poverty, in a world where long-standing value commitments are weakening, both within the profession and within society as a whole. It concludes by establishing the relationship between tackling exclusion and social justice. Chapter 3 considers the building blocks for tackling exclusion.

The volume then shifts gear by looking at practice as it relates to specific groups of users. Chapter 4 considers work with socially excluded children and families – children in need, children with disabilities, so-called 'troubled' families. Chapter 5 considers work with excluded young people – those engaging in anti-social behaviour and care leavers for example. Chapter 6 examines work with socially excluded adults in a fast-fragmenting adult social care environment. It pays particular attention to community-level initiatives in combating, for example, loneliness in old age.

Chapter 7 looks at how entire communities and neighbourhoods become excluded, before it suggests ways to tackle this disadvantage at a community level. Chapter 8 examines the particular characteristics of social exclusion in rural areas and the difficulties that they present practitioners working in rural communities. Chapter 9 addresses racism, immigration and asylum. The final chapter discusses how organisations learn about justice through evaluation, and what are the possible foundational concepts that can tie social work practice to social justice aims for the next decade.

CHAPTER 1

WHAT SOCIAL EXCLUSION MEANS

THIS CHAPTER COVERS

- Evolution of social exclusion as a concept.

- The components of exclusion: poverty, failure in the job market, poorly performing social networks, living in a disadvantaged neighbourhood, and exclusion from services.

- An understanding of what social exclusion means for social work practice and why tackling it is a key task in the pursuit of a fairer society.

Social exclusion, as a concept, captures the process through which people's lives are shaped by multiple disadvantages without the material and social resources most of us take for granted. While we can roughly estimate the number of people socially excluded – and particularly whether that number is increasing or decreasing – that is not the major purpose of the concept for social workers. Rather it enables social workers to understand how need, deprivation, loneliness, poverty and poor health combine in ways that affect individuals, families and neighbourhoods both materially and psychologically. In a profession overly prone to assigning people to separate categories according to eligibility criteria, social exclusion requires us to look at a person or family as a product of social and economic forces as well as of individual motivation, upbringing and culture. While social work theory has long stressed the 'person in their environment', social exclusion gives us a concrete account of how this happens – uncovering processes and categories that link the thinking and behaviour of users to their social conditions.

How and why people are excluded is a sharply contested question with views running across a spectrum. At one end are those who see the exclusion of the individual as entirely their own responsibility – and therefore solutions are to do with correcting individual behaviour and beliefs. At the other end are those who regard the behaviour of excluded individuals as a product of large-scale economic structures and social forces over which they have little control. Of course a substantial middle part of the spectrum blends together some ideas from each of these extremes, while social policy of central government bends first one way and then the other. This debate, which has been with us in one form or another since the dawn of industrialisation in the early 1800s, continues to impact on social policy and on social work.

EVOLUTION OF A CONCEPT

Social exclusion has been succinctly defined as 'chronic, multidimensional disadvantage resulting in a catastrophic detachment from society' (Burchardt *et al.* 1999). It affects key domains of family and community life – health, child development, educational attainment, nutrition, parenting skills, household income and participation in the labour market. The concept helps us identify and investigate these separate dimensions and then to see how they reinforce each other in the lives of those social workers mainly work with.

Despite the various meanings that social exclusion has acquired in recent years in Britain, the concept itself arose in a specific context in France in the 1970s. There it was used to describe the condition of certain groups on the margins of society who were cut off both from regular sources of employment *and* the income safety nets of the welfare state. *Les exclus* lacked the substantial rights of *les citoyens*, either in practice, because they were victims of discrimination such as disabled people, or because they were not citizens of the state, such as immigrants. Nor did they have access to or connections with those powerful institutions that might have helped them gain voice such as the trade unions or residents' associations.

It is important to remember that the concept of social exclusion arose in France and not in Britain or the United States, both of which have substantially different political cultures in which there is a higher tolerance for inequality and the expansion of the free market in delivering public services. The idea of social 'solidarity' from which social exclusion emerged was and remains an important element in the French Republican ideal and very different from the tradition of investigation begun by Charles Booth and Seebohm Rowntree on the poverty line and numbers falling below it. Drawing on this ideal was the means by which the French state could repair the rupture of the social fabric rather than through sociological analysis of the incidence of poverty. Social solidarity required an emphasis on citizenship and social cohesion, reflecting a strong state with a commitment to providing a social safety net for those outside the labour market (Paugam 1993).

From France the term gained wide currency in the social policy of the European Union, particularly in the Maastricht Treaty of 1996. Conservatives on the right supported it because it did not necessarily focus only on poverty and income, while the social democratic left saw it as a way of promoting inclusion and social justice.

Tackling exclusion and promoting inclusion gained wide appeal across the political spectrum. For the political left it suggested a greater push toward equality with a focus on tackling deprivation and the lack of rights, while for the right it suggested shaping a more cohesive, unified society uniting behind a strong national regime. For the right, wanting to back away from the anti-poverty strategies of the 1960s and 1970s that had focused on improving welfare benefits, the concept gave government room to look more closely at individual attributes such as resilience, motivation, work discipline and parenting skills as among the causes of poverty. This was indeed one of its attractions as a policy tool – it enabled politicians and policy makers to move from focusing only on income to the interaction between behaviour and economic necessity.

When the Labour Party came to power in the UK in 1997 it swiftly adopted the concept as its own, framing a range of social policy objectives in terms of reducing social exclusion. It set up the Social Exclusion Unit in the Cabinet Office to ensure that all departments coordinated their efforts in tackling exclusion. This in turn was replaced in 2004 by the Social Exclusion Task Force, still within the Cabinet Office, as government recognised that it had to restructure its inclusion policies to focus on chronically excluded adults and multi-problem families.

In its transition from continental Europe to the UK, social exclusion became more flexible as a policy vehicle, incorporating earlier strands of welfare policy in the UK, such as raising levels of benefits, along with newer elements such as placing some conditions on receiving those benefits. Yet the importance of what was new should not be underestimated. Using social exclusion as the focal point for policy marked a profound break with government philosophy of the two decades from the mid-1970s to the mid-1990s. During this period Britain not only saw a large rise in the proportion of its people living in poverty, particularly children, but had the fastest rate of rising inequality in the world, with the exception of New Zealand. Even so, Conservative ministers had from time to time suggested there was no such thing as poverty in Britain. From 1997 on, the British government at least recognised that exclusion undermined social and individual wellbeing to an unacceptable degree and announced its intention to do something about it.

That social exclusion means different things to different people is part of its appeal and effectiveness in formulating policy and practice. But its multiple meanings also present conceptual difficulty for as soon as a discussion of social exclusion gets underway, contentious issues arise, principally because people with different points of view find different meanings in the concept. At stake are deeply held values about society and the causes of social problems. Some of the differing viewpoints include:

- As a concept social exclusion is overly vague and appeals to those who would prefer not to think about poverty. The European Union has used it for this reason – it allows governments to reconcile a bland notion of social justice with high levels of inequality and dispossession.
- People exclude themselves from mainstream society. They do this through their own irresponsible choices and lack of willingness to participate in the labour market, and hence become dependent on benefits.
- Work is the most effective way of overcoming social exclusion because it provides social connections and higher levels of income than benefits. Welfare policy therefore should contain forceful encouragement and even compulsion for all on benefits – including disabled people and lone mothers – to take on paid employment.
- Focusing on poverty means only looking at income as the basis for quality of life; social exclusion by contrast focuses more on social relations and the extent to

which people are able to participate in social affairs and attain sufficient power to influence decisions that affect them.

Each of the above points has those who agree and disagree with it. For example, on the third point, disabled people and their advocates and representatives strongly contest the fact that they are compelled to attend medical examinations which find them 'work ready', with the attendant pressure that they should find a job, when in fact they face discrimination and barriers to the workplace. The problem, they argue, lies not with disabled people but in the labour market, which is dominated by exclusionary practices in relation to people with disability and workplaces with poor access. They argue that many of the forces of exclusion lie outside the individual's capacity to act. Those who argue for the second point, that social exclusion is a consequence of individual habits and personality, maintain that overcoming exclusion lies in the individual's capacity to change.

It is difficult to resolve these questions one way or another, simply because they call on different and opposing sets of values. Even so, as practitioners accumulate experience they will begin to develop their own understanding of the causes of exclusion, of what the experience of exclusion is like, what defines it and the ways in which they may be able to counter it.

MAKING SENSE OF SOCIAL EXCLUSION

Since the late nineteenth century social investigators have regarded poverty as an objective, quantifiable condition, one that can be measured against a calculated standard: the poverty line. Largely developed within an Anglo-American tradition of empiricism the concept of the poverty line was used to determine eligibility for poor relief and as a prod for social policy to do more. Poverty was no longer seen as a natural phenomenon but could be explained and reduced by rational policies (O'Connor 2001: 14). Alongside this approach however was a contrary one, more deeply embedded in governments and in the popular mind, that poverty is a product of dysfunction, deviance or the self-perpetuating 'tangle of pathology'. In this account, poverty is a product of individual character and behaviour, of psychological and cultural practices that are resistant to, and even take advantage of, state-provided poverty relief programmes.

Social exclusion, as a concept, can best be understood as trying to bridge the gap between these two contrary approaches, at once able to shed light on structural causes of poverty – low wages, economic disorganisation, discrimination – and on its cultural, moral and behavioural sources. Elasticity is built into the concept for this very reason; its objective is to define a number of factors, both individual and familial as well as social and economic, to account for the extent of poverty in a society *and* the psychological disengagement, alienation, that is its by-product. The kinds of solutions proposed to overcome exclusion are not only economic but seek to re-establish social solidarity, social cohesion.

In an influential text of the late 1990s, Ruth Levitas noted three different political discourses within the concept of social exclusion:

- A *redistributionist* discourse, which she codenamed RED, that advocated income transfers through tax and benefits from wealthier households to low-income households and neighbourhoods.

- A *social integrationist* discourse, codenamed SID, that first and foremost sought social cohesion and regarded social exclusion as a divisive force which, if left unchecked, created dangerous divisions within a society.
- A *moral underclass* discourse, codenamed MUD, that viewed social exclusion as a matter of individual responsibility arising from poor character and poor life choices.

(Levitas 2005)

Levitas neatly summarised the contradictory perspectives that social exclusion embraced at that time. What has changed since then is the balance of influence among these three discourses. Whereas in the early years of New Labour it was possible to say that the redistributionist policies overlapped with social integration policies to form the New Labour project (working families tax credits, Sure Start programmes in disadvantaged neighbourhoods, neighbourhood renewal programmes, Health Action Zones, community cohesion policies – all brought about some transfer of resources to low-income families and neighbourhoods), in the later years of the Labour administration, that balance had begun to change, with greater focus on the behaviour of problem families, tighter conditions for receiving benefits, coaching individuals to become more work ready – policies that leaned more toward the moral underclass perspective.

But that change was small compared to the changing fortunes of the three discourses following the 'austerity' election of 2010 when the redistributionist discourse – reducing income inequality through taxes and benefits – lost all its persuasiveness within central government. By contrast, as noted in the introduction to this volume, the underclass discourse, once confined to the extreme right wing throughout the 1970s, 1980s and 1990s, thrived at the Department for Work and Pensions and underpinned the radical overhaul of the benefits system under the Coalition and Conservative governments from 2010 on (HM Government 2012).

From its first formulations, then, there was a fundamental ambiguity in the term 'social exclusion' which referred to those in poverty and the long-term unemployed but also to those who did not fit into society, with tacit acknowledgement that behaviour was part of the problem. The ambiguities of social exclusion arise precisely because it is a concept that spans a number of domains – the impact of social and economic structures on individuals, families and neighbourhoods as well as the domains of behaviour and cultural and moral values. This is its strength – it potentially offers a holistic conceptualisation of disadvantage as a phenomenon constructed by interlocking forces from within those domains. This is also its weakness – it is a highly elastic concept, vulnerable to specific, ideologically guided interpretations that, while employing the phrase, implicitly leave behind ecological and whole-systems thinking to settle on particular parts of the system: the rigidity of public service bureaucracies for example or the behaviour of 'hard to reach' families.

MONITORING SOCIAL EXCLUSION ANNUALLY

The New Policy Institute reviews the extent of social exclusion each year using the same set of indicators to allow year-on-year comparison. These indicators help clarify the kinds of circumstances that contribute to social exclusion. Some of the indicators are:

Money: percentage of children in poverty, number of workless families in poverty, number of working families in poverty, poverty among families with disabled people;

Housing: number of housing benefit claimants, overcrowding among renting households, number of social housing renters in poverty;

Work: number of people underemployed and unemployed, number of involuntary temporary employees, number of long-term unemployed;

Benefits: value of means-tested benefits; number of Job Seeker's Allowance (JSA) claimants, number of sanctions on those receiving JSA.

(MacInnes *et al.* 2014)

Indicators have great value in pointing to the extent of exclusion but they do not provide a complete representation of what it means to be excluded. They are simply an *indication*, as their name suggests. They help enlarge our understanding of exclusion but do not provide an immediate explanation of it.

This ambiguity raised the conceptual difficulty of distinguishing 'poverty' from 'social exclusion' – the two concepts are so entwined that in much social policy and research parlance the two are linked together in a single phrase. There is no 'social exclusion line' as there is a 'poverty line' but as social exclusion began to attract wider attention among policy circles and poverty researchers, attempts were made to pin down formally what defined it. Definitions were never more than approximate. They commonly stressed: (i) the multi-dimensional nature of exclusion – social, economic and psychological; (ii) the *relational* nature of exclusion and the subjective, felt experience of those excluded, in the form of social distance, humiliation, shame, rejection, not being able to participate; (iii) that exclusion was *relative* to the society within which it took place; (iv) the dynamic nature of exclusion – how it is self-reinforcing, tends to perpetuate itself and be resistant to measures to combat it (Atkinson 2002; Silver and Miller 2004; Burchardt 1999).

REFLECT AND DECIDE: WHAT CAUSES POVERTY?

Iain Duncan Smith, Secretary of State, Department for Work and Pensions, spoke on welfare reform on 23 January 2014:

> for most people, their life's direction of travel is dictated by the informed decisions they make: can they afford a large family . . . should they move in order to take up a better-paid job . . . can they risk a mortgage to get a bigger home? Yet, too often for those locked in the benefits system, that process of making responsible and positive choices has been skewed – money paid out to pacify them regardless, with no incentive to aspire for a better life.

According to the minister, what is the reason that people find themselves in poverty? What is the effect of the benefits system on human behaviour? What does he mean by 'pacify'? Do benefits dampen aspiration? What other interpretations of the causes of poverty are possible?

A BROAD DEFINITION OF SOCIAL EXCLUSION

Reflecting the broad nature of social exclusion, definitions generally attempt to high-light the causes of exclusion in ways that enable analysis of the interaction of its different aspects in relation to individuals, families and neighbourhoods (Burchardt *et al.* 2002: 7).

With fundamental arguments over human behaviour at stake it is not surprising that reaching a single, reliable definition of social exclusion in practice is difficult. The viewpoint offered in this volume places a greater weight on poverty as the principal but not exclusive shaper of human behaviour, rather than such factors as individual motivation, moral capacity or personality characteristics. Poverty drastically reduces the range of choices that individuals and families have at their disposal. What appear as reasonable, responsible courses of action for individuals and families are often simply not available to those below the poverty line, because access to resources, the means, the knowledge and the support, which others take for granted, are not there. Poverty, then, is a kind of ultimate indicator, signalling that some people are on the receiving end of broad social and economic inequalities.

In any definition of social exclusion, participation in society at large is central. What exactly is to be participated in is always up for further discussion – but as a gen-eralisation it refers to participation in the normal, everyday activities of citizens and residents *when the excluded want to do so but are prevented by factors beyond their control* (Burchardt *et al.* 1999). The emphasis here is that a person (or indeed family or neighbourhood) is excluded through circumstances not of their own making – in other words individuals cannot exclude themselves through their own behaviour (Burchardt *et al.* 2002: 30).

CASE STUDIES IN EXCLUSION

(1)   Max is 7 with autism. He is the youngest of five, and at school he shows disruptive behaviour on occasion. The other four children are 13 and up and attend high school. His mother, Maryanne, 36, lives in privately rented accommodation with her children on the edge of a medium-sized town in a largely rural county borough. She has no partner. Maryanne does not work and is regularly asked by Jobcentre Plus staff to attend a work readiness interview. She lives week to week on child benefit, housing benefit and job seeker's allowance.

(2)   Mrs W, age 56, has multiple sclerosis and is short of breath. She used to work as a health therapist but no long can because of her condition. She is divorced with two sons living a considerable distance away. She has a small personal network of friends. Previously she had a personal budget to pay for her care but she has so far been unable to find the right carer. Her illness has recently progressed and the local authority has asked her to complete a self-assessment of needs with support from one of her sons.

(3)   A large disadvantaged housing estate lies on the edge of Leeds with clearly demar-cated geographical and transport boundaries that separate it from the city. The estate

was built in the 1940s to replace housing lost during World War II. A large part of the population live below the poverty line. Over two-thirds of households in the area live in social housing; there is a noticeable polarisation of age of residents – older people who have lived there for decades and younger single-parent families who are recent arrivals. Migrants from Europe and asylum seekers are also housed on the estate. A dispersal order – that is a measure that empowers local police to disperse groups of young people in order to prevent anti-social behaviour – has been granted to cover most of the estate. Now when some residents see groups of young people gathering they ring the police who respond quickly to break the groups up.

Each of the above are excluded in different ways. In reflecting on their circumstances and the ways in which they are excluded, consider the different components that make up exclusion: income, disability or chronic sickness, responsiveness (or not) of services, the extent of social networks, access to the job market, and overall neighbourhood environment. Of course only scanty information is provided for each here – but these short summaries can be mapped on to more detailed account of users' lives with the aim of getting you to think about the components of exclusion with those you work with.

What of individual motivation, individual choices and behaviour? Are people not also responsible for excluding themselves – for example by criminal or anti-social behaviour, or wilful neglect of children? The question lies at the heart of political differences. How much for example does disadvantage shape an individual's behaviour and choices, despite that individual's best efforts – and how much is due to wilful, wrong-headed choices that arise wholly within an individual's own decision-making process? Take for example joblessness: does it run in families? The political right says yes, it is a culture passed across generations. Other researchers who have conducted longitudinal studies on joblessness say yes, it is intergenerational but there are deeper reasons for this than an individual family's culture: for example a depressed labour market in a locality that has lost its manufacturing base and where job opportunities are scarce (Tilly 1998; Feinstein *et al.* 2008).

The terms right and left refer to positional attitudes on the political spectrum. The notion of 'the left' as the more radical position developed simply because during the French Revolution of 1789 the factions that sat to the left of the speaker in the national assembly were the more radical groupings, while those on the right were the more conservative. The terms have stuck and are relevant to the debate over the causes of poverty and social exclusion.

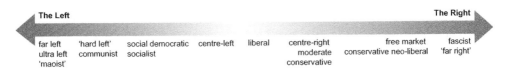

FIGURE 1.1   The political spectrum: an overview (author)

Reflecting the multi-dimensional nature of social exclusion we adopt the following definition:

> Social exclusion is a process over time that deprives individuals and families, groups and neighbourhoods of the resources required for participation in the social, economic and political activity of society as a whole. This process is primarily a consequence of poverty and low income, but other factors such as discrimination, low educational attainment and depleted environments also underpin it. Through this process people are cut off for a significant period in their lives from institutions and services, social networks and developmental opportunities that the great majority of a society enjoy.

COMPONENTS OF SOCIAL EXCLUSION

We have thus far discussed the tensions within the concept of social exclusion, have begun to think about what being socially excluded actually means for people and have formulated a working definition of social exclusion as a process that extends over time. This section follows up by examining the five main components that drive this process:

- poverty and low income
- lack of access to the jobs market
- social isolation and failure of social networks
- neighbourhood disadvantage and the effects on those living there
- exclusion from services.

Poverty and low income

The definition acknowledges that poverty is a potent exclusionary force. Any social work practice that aims to reduce exclusion cannot avoid this central fact. Often 'poverty and social exclusion' are linked to ensure that this is understood. Indeed a family with a reasonable income, or a local neighbourhood with reasonable median income, will usually have ready resources – from social networks to educational attainments to funding local community initiatives – to overcome barriers and exclusions that they may encounter. On the other hand, those without material resources, those who have a continuous shortfall of income, not only have to go without certain necessities but also experience emotional and psychological challenges that those above the poverty line do not face.

The sociologist Peter Townsend is largely credited with developing a multi-dimensional approach to poverty, a forerunner to the concept of social exclusion. Poverty in Townsend's view is *relative*, that is, people are poor in relation to the society in which they live. He wrote in 1962: 'Society itself is continuously changing and thrusting new obligations on its members. They in turn develop new needs' (Townsend 1962: 225). And in his great work on poverty he wrote: 'Individuals, families and groups . . . can be said to be in poverty when they lack the resources to obtain the types of diet, participate in the activities and have the living conditions and amenities which are customary . . . in the societies in which they belong' (Townsend 1979: 31). In pursuing this, Townsend drew up an index of living standards, including diet, clothing, recreation and household amenities, with the aim of linking levels of income to whether these items were obtainable or not. Ultimately Townsend did relate income to the ability to purchase these items and in that sense defined poverty in terms of income alone (Mack *et al.* 2013).

MEASURING INCOME

The most commonly used measure for determining income poverty is whether household income falls below 60 per cent of household median income. The standard is used throughout the EU: incomes below that standard are insufficient to obtain the necessities and resources for participation in society. The advantage of using median income – the midpoint of all household incomes with as many above as below the median – is that, unlike average or 'mean' income, it is unaffected by changes in the incomes of the very wealthy and is therefore a better indicator of what is considered normal in society at large.

Indicators of social exclusion move beyond focusing on income alone to highlight the lack of societal participation, as Townsend foreshadowed. The proliferation of different poverty measures and indicators can be confusing, with no single set of indicators universally accepted. However, important work has been done linking measures of poverty to the various ways people are cut off from, denied, or cannot take part in or enjoy the advantages of common social engagement. This is the major contribution of social exclusion as a concept: to link lack of income to *the ways in which people are unable to exert influence over the institutions that shape their lives.*

Mack and Lansley have been charting what the public considers a minimum standard of living that enables a person to have a certain number of basic necessities. Their studies use a measure of poverty which is based on a consensus of what the public deems as necessary to achieve a basic level of wellbeing. Over a thirty-year period they have found widespread agreement across all groups in society – whether by gender, age, occupation, income level, geography or even political views – about the relative importance of different items and activities. One of their most important findings was that the public itself has a relativist view of poverty, with its definition of what is necessary for a minimum standard going beyond basic physiological need to reflect contemporary living standards – at its core it should enable a person to take part in the society in which they live (Mack and Lansley 2012). Their latest survey in 2012 only underpins this consistency of viewpoint. They conclude that the public believes that a minimum standard is not simply about subsistence, but should reflect contemporary standards sufficient to enable people to participate fully in the society in which they live.

THE PUBLIC'S VIEW OF A MINIMUM STANDARD OF LIVING

The most heavily supported items relate to what traditionally have been seen as basic needs – shelter, food and clothing. In the Mack and Lansley survey, 96 per cent of the public thought people should have sufficient income to heat the living areas of the home, 94 per cent to keep their home damp-free, and 91 per cent to have two meals a day. Income enough to visit friends or family in hospital or other institutions had slightly less public support at 90 per cent; celebrations on special occasions 80 per cent; attendance at weddings, funerals and other such occasions 79 per cent.

For children, the public are more generous than with adults. The top four items are: a warm winter coat, 97 per cent; fresh fruit and vegetables once a day, 96 per cent; new, properly fitting shoes, 93 per cent; three meals a day, 93 per cent; celebrations on special occasions, 91 per cent; hobbies or leisure activities, 88 per cent; toddler groups or nursery or play group at least once a week for pre-school-aged children, 87 per cent; children's clubs or activities such as drama or football training, 74 per cent (Mack and Lansley 2012).

Poverty and personal distress

The pain of poverty extends beyond material hardship. For all the efforts to define poverty around its economic consequences it is the experience of being poor and the loss of self-respect that drives a wedge between those below the minimum standard and the rest. The Nobel-winning economist Amartya Sen has said that we should not just focus on low income itself but also on psychological effects of being poor, on 'the feelings of deprivation' that low income produces (Sen 1982). Although the poor are sometimes portrayed as shameless in their apparent willingness to accept welfare benefits and their chaotic lifestyles, the opposite is the case: poor people feel ashamed at not being able to fulfil their personal aspirations or to live up to societal expectations due to their lack of income and other resources. Poverty then is not just learning to go without, but has emotional, psychological consequences – the loss of self-belief and dignity from being unable to participate in society as others do.

Shame lies at the 'irreducible absolutist core' of poverty (Sen 1983: 159, cited in Walker 2014: 65). The shame of being poor is externally imposed by society through those institutions and individuals motivated to engage in shaming, but is internalised as a powerful emotion leading to social withdrawal and a sense of powerlessness (see Figure 1.2). Should the poor

> fail to appreciate the degree of their inadequacy and the depth of their degradation, society takes it upon itself to shame them into changing their ways or, with similar intent, to stigmatize them, thereby reinforcing social divisions of 'us' and 'them' and often actively discriminating against the them, 'the poor'.
>
> (Walker 2014: 65)

One of the Coalition's policy objectives was to enshrine this process in law, with powerful ripple effects throughout the media and public attitudes.

GENDER AND POVERTY STATISTICS

Poverty and social exclusion indicators can easily overlook women when reporting on patterns of household income and consumption. Poverty statistics when considering consumption or income tend to treat the household as a sharing unit. This conceals significant inequalities between women and men in control over resources and the question of who does what labour within the household. As a consequence, statistics and indicators often seriously underestimate the extent to which poverty is feminised.

Living on a low income, under conditions of scarcity, a person only focuses on expenses that are staring them in the face. The person in poverty draws on future resources – as limited as they might be – in order to navigate through the day. A similar pressure exists in relation to time. When people are short of time, having to execute trade-offs between today and tomorrow, they are doing something very similar to juggling their finances. 'It is all scarcity juggling. You borrow from tomorrow, and tomorrow you have less time than you have today, and tomorrow becomes more costly. It's a very costly loan' (Mullainathan and Shafir 2014). Richard Sennett notes that in formation of character, inequality 'translates into doubt of self' to the point that one is 'not seen' (Sennett 1998: 3), restricting the feeling of being able to influence the views and behaviour of other people, particularly in challenging bureaucratic systemic structures that coerce and intervene in their lives (ibid.: 21).

CHARLES BLOW ON POVERTY

Poverty is a demanding, stressful, depressive and often violent state. No one seeks it; they are born or thrust into it. In poverty, the whole of your life becomes an exercise in coping and correcting, searching for a way up and out, while focusing today on filling the pots and the plates, maintaining a roof and some warmth, and dreading the new challenge tomorrow may bring.

(Blow 2014)

In general social scientists argue that the greater the degree of inequality within a society the less cohesive and less productive that society will be. Income inequality is a powerful social divider and living standards are markers of difference in status. Where we are in the social hierarchy affects who is the in-group and who is out-group – us and them – undermining our ability to identify with and empathise with other people (Wilkinson and Pickett 2010: 51). Michael Sandel put it this way: 'In a society where every thing is for sale, life is harder for those of modest means. The more money can buy the more affluence (or lack of it) matters' (Sandel 2013: 8).

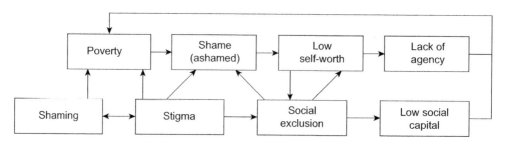

FIGURE 1.2   Walker's model of poverty and shame (Walker 2014; reproduced with permission
from Oxford University Press)

Access to the jobs market and paid employment

Work – aspiring toward it, finding it, keeping it, getting paid for it – is the main
objective of Conservative social policy. Indeed for adults of working age (and their
dependants), whatever their needs, the labour market can now be deemed the central
institution through which welfare is channelled. The central, but hidden, conflict is
between conceptualisations of human need and the demands of the labour market. The
welfare state as classically conceived was to shield people who could not participate
in the labour market or, because of injury, health or incapacity, were kept from participating in the labour market. In this sense the welfare state 'decommodified' people,
as social scientists put it, shielding them and their dependants from becoming a pure
human commodity within the labour market.

Now, under welfare reform, the conflict between human need and being 'work-
ready' is played out within individual lives in the context of labour market demands.
Indeed human need is defined not in opposition to the labour market but *only* in terms
of what is required to allow a person to enter the labour market. Of course, while
legislation can narrow the concept of human need in this way, actual need, of lone
parents, of children in poverty, of those with disability and the long-term sick, does
not disappear. Social workers' role often lies in bridging this gap between need defined
as deficits in relation to the labour market and need defined as elements of self-respect,
dignity and wellbeing.

Absence of social networks and social supports

A third component of social exclusion is the weakness in social networks. 'Network
poverty' deprives users of friendships, social contact and informal help that we all draw
on to participate in community life and to enjoy the standards of living shared by the
majority of people. Social work has formally acknowledged this to be the case for some
while. For example, since the implementation of the Children Act 1989 the official preference is to place children with relatives and as near to home as possible rather than in
a children's home or with distant foster parents, thus preserving the child's familial and
social contacts. In general, practitioner focus on networks has been intermittent and
often of low priority. For instance in social care for older people social workers have

reduced their engagement with 'non-care' activities such as developing luncheon clubs, providing specialist transport services and befriending activities, which has undermined the network-enhancing role of social care practice, leaving those functions to local voluntary groups. This is despite the clear evidence that networks and neighbourhood involvement are instrumental in underpinning older people's wellbeing (Wenger 1997; McLeod 2008; see Chapter 7).

Loneliness and isolation

Loneliness, it has been found, adversely affects both physical and mental health, particularly among older adults, and has been compared in harm to the damaging health effects of smoking and other major risks (Hemingway and Jack 2013). Loneliness stems in part from the way in which a person experiences and evaluates his or her isolation and absence of communication with other people. It is this subjective element that makes it possible for a person to be isolated without feeling lonely, and to feel lonely without being isolated.

Loneliness varies with age – but not necessarily in ways that you would think. For example, a survey from the Mental Health Foundation suggests that loneliness is more prevalent than expected among young people, with some 60 per cent between the ages of 18 and 34 in the survey reporting feeling lonely often or sometimes. Loneliness also poses a particular threat to the very old, with evidence pointing to cognitive decline and shortened lives of those that are lonely (Mental Health Foundation 2013). In one well-known experiment ten volunteers aged 22 to 50 spent a week wearing gloves and vision-impairing glasses to mimic the effects of ageing, and only had a television for company. They struggled to cope without human contact for a week as part of a social experiment and within three to five days many participants started to feel desperate (Anonymous 2011).

REFLECT AND DECIDE: WHAT CAUSES LONELINESS?

Surveys regularly record an increase in loneliness within society. By way of explanation some argue that we have become more self-centred as individuals, less inclined to contribute to a wider collective, and even less inclined to establish and deeply commit to individual relationships. Is this the backdrop to increasing loneliness?

Disadvantaged neighbourhoods

Since the 1990s we have learned an immense amount about the power of 'place' – the impact of neighbourhood on the lives of those that live there. We know that conditions of poverty and exclusion interact and reinforce each other in particular geographical locations to create a qualitatively different set of conditions that make it virtually impossible for individuals or families to escape these negative 'neighbourhood' effects.

This dynamic between poor schooling, vulnerable families and low income is found throughout the UK, often on social housing estates on the edges of towns and cities, but also in low-income areas of mixed tenancy and owner-occupied housing in both urban and rural neighbourhoods.

In disadvantaged neighbourhoods various components of exclusion reinforce each other so that everyone in that particular area is affected. Services have been withdrawn, fear of crime is high, levels of political participation low. Employers and commercial outlets have left the area, taking jobs with them. Without the resources from effective services, wages from steady employment, and support networks based on reasonable levels of trust, the neighbourhood stressors mount up on children, parents and vulnerable adults alike. When an entire neighbourhood is excluded, such as a social housing estate, the most damaging long-term impact arises from what sociologists call 'neighbourhood effects' – the decline in the social fabric and loss of control over public space that affect the quality of life of all residents in a particular area regardless of individual levels of aspiration or motivation.

Many of these effects on individual behaviour profoundly impact on social work. For example, child outcomes such as infant mortality and low birth weight have been tied to neighbourhood disadvantage; so have rates of teenage pregnancy and school exclusion; while child abuse and neglect and anti-social behaviour by young people have all been linked to living in neighbourhoods with particular characteristics (Brooks-Gunn *et al.* 1997); so has accidental injury to children and the suicide of young people (Almgren in Sampson *et al.* 2002).

A link between the prevalence of crime within neighbourhoods and the 'efficacy' of neighbourhoods, that is the effectiveness with which social norms are projected and protected in public spaces, is also well established (Sampson *et al.* 2002). Neighbourhood environments contribute to the inequalities in health, with chronic disease, such as obesity and diabetes, and mental health problems, such as depression and anxiety, more prevalent in disadvantaged neighbourhoods (Diez Rous and Mair 2010).

Where ethnic minorities are concentrated in relatively deprived urban areas, employment prospects are affected, with, for example, higher rates of unemployment and lower rates of self-employment than ethnically balanced areas (Clark and Drinkwater 2002). A profound negative effect on the emotional stability of pre-school children exposed to neighbourhood violence has been established (Farver and Natera 2000). Neighbourhoods impact on a range of health outcomes, including low birth weight, attitudes to nutrition and exercise, levels of adult mortality, cardiovascular risk factors and many others (Diez-Roux 2001; Acheson 1998; Browning and Cagney 2002).

The neighbourhood as the focus for combating exclusion is not the rosy world of mutual help evoked in memoirs of working-class urban districts (Roberts 1973; Woodruff 2002) and Welsh mining communities, or in the idyllic pictures of suburban living in the 1950s. Today when we talk of neighbourhood we may mean nothing more than an area with some sense of physical boundary or other defining limits. In tackling exclusion, neighbourhoods become the focus, not because of any belief in a false consensus but because local areas are sites where multiple strands of exclusion come together. In fact practitioners will want to ensure that they uncover any false consensus and recognise local diversity, whether in culture, ethnicity, gender or income levels.

The most disadvantaged neighbourhoods in Britain are generally found in inner-city social housing flats such as high rises, the decaying owner-occupied or privately rented terraced housing of older cities, and the peripheral housing estates that ring many of

Britain's urban areas. Even prosperous towns have large council-owned estates that over a period of time have experienced intense deprivation. The overall impact of disadvantage is that residents do not see themselves as being in control; what they want is to have influence over regular services rather than special projects. Yet neighbourhoods do matter to their residents, and it is wrong to simply assume that disadvantaged areas totally lack social cohesion or are empty of support networks and people with skills and talent.

Many 'high unemployment' neighbourhoods have remained continuously disadvantaged over decades. Of the 600 communities in the top 10 per cent in England for unemployment in 2009, three-quarters were in the top 10 per cent in 2005 when unemployment was much lower, and nearly half had been in the top 10 per cent in boom and bust since 1985 (Tunstall 2009: 4). Palmer *et al.* (2006) found similar results, using a broader measure of all benefits claims against micro neighbourhood data known as 'super output areas' (slightly smaller than postcode sectors). They found that, of the areas in the top decile for benefits receipt in 1999, 86 per cent were still in the top tenth in 2005, six years later.

Exclusion from services

Lack of access to services is the fifth and final component of exclusion. By 'services' we mean the whole range of private and public, in-home and out-of-home services that individuals, families and groups continually draw on for a variety of purposes. In-home services include everything from electricity to care for those who need it; out-of-home services include transport, post office, banking, doctor and hospital facilities, or those such as day care for children and day centres for older people. In poor or disadvantaged neighbourhoods there are often barriers to obtaining such services beyond the means of any one individual or family to surmount. They may be remote in style, reliant on jargon, difficult to access by public transport; others may have points for local contact but may be poor in quality, lacking in privacy, or have tough eligibility criteria.

One national example of service withdrawal is the decrease in use of community services by those over 65. The number of older people using day-care centres fell by 49 percent – from 136,000 to 69,100 between 2006 and 2013. The proportion of older people receiving home care also fell by 21 per cent during that same period. (By contrast older people using residential care homes rose 21 per cent while those using nursing care rose by 22 per cent – a sharp reversal of community care policy.) In 2011, out of an estimated 2 million older people with care-related needs, some 800,000 received no support from public or private sector agencies (Age UK 2014). The reasons behind this fall are not hard to find – councils received less funding from central government and home care is high on the list for council cuts.

Another very different example is found in the exclusion that lesbian, gay, bisexual and transgender young people often experience in school through the combined impact of institutional ignorance and dominant heterosexual assumptions. Bullying and name calling by other pupils such as 'tranny' or 'man-beast', and being spat on or attacked in corridors provide daily threats and fear of violence that completes the sense of ostracism.

SOCIAL WORK AND SOCIAL EXCLUSION

Does social exclusion change the way in which social work views its practice, or has it simply re-cast long-recognised problems in a new language without offering any new ideas on how to tackle them? The concept extends practitioner understanding of three domains in users' lives: participation and engagement in society, the multi-dimensionality of poverty, and a better understanding of 'agency' – the extent to which a person can function effectively in their social environment. For example, social exclusion draws specific attention to the extent to which a child engages with peers, and, conversely, highlights the barriers faced by excluded children, such as educational difficulties, poor health, anti-social behaviour. Axford contrasts an approach based on social exclusion with a 'needs' approach typically expressed in terms of health and development. The first suggests strengthening a child's capacity to join and integrate with others, while the second requires that the child must show actual or likely impairment to health or development to be deemed 'in need'. There is tension between the two: the one maximises inclusion, the other minimises harm (Axford 2010: 738).

There are, however, tendencies inherent in the way the social exclusion perspective is used that can render it less radical than some advocates would prefer (Morris and Barnes 2008: 267), with a drift towards a 'weak' model of exclusion focused on the excluded individual, and away from the 'strong' model with its emphasis on institutions and economic structures in the exclusion process.

The tension within the concept – locating the causes of poverty and durable inequalities in social structures or within individual behaviour – is not as sharp in practice as in theoretical debates. Blau's (1960) essential insight still holds: that structural effects operate through, and in concert with, individual effects. Social workers work with individuals and on a day-to-day basis they do not get near the big levers that would significantly improve users' resources collectively, such as expanding low-rent housing, lowering the cost of child care, improving the quality of the local school, building a play

REFLECT AND DECIDE: WHAT CAN SOCIAL WORK DO ABOUT SOCIAL EXCLUSION?

The list of social problems that the Social Exclusion Task Force (2004) associated with exclusion is long: lack of opportunities for work, lack of opportunities to acquire education and work-related skills, childhood deprivation, families disrupted through high levels of conflict, separation or divorce, barriers to older people living active lives, inequalities in health, poor housing, poor neighbourhoods, fear of crime, and groups disadvantaged through poverty or discrimination.

Think of your current set of job or placement responsibilities and decide which of the social problems listed above you and your team could tackle. You might want to categorise those problems according to whether you and your team's job specifications would have scope for tackling those problems on your own or in collaboration with other organisations. If you are a social work or social care student, pick out those skills and competencies that you think could be applied to reducing the exclusion of various service user groups.

park for children, supplying more free hours of adult social care. But a social exclusion perspective points them to other means that can disrupt or soften structural impacts. One of these, noted throughout the book, is to look for community-level solutions in which participation and user engagement become prominent.

KEY POINTS

❑   Social exclusion is a process that deprives individuals, families, groups and neighbourhoods of the resources for participation in social, economic and political activity that the great majority of society enjoys. These resources are not just material but have to do with the quality of social interaction. Social exclusion undermines or destroys channels of access for support and opportunity. It brings with it a sense of shame and loss of dignity and therefore has profound psychological and emotional consequences.

❑   The five main strands of social exclusion are: (i) poverty and low income; (ii) barriers to the jobs market; (iii) lack of social networks; (iv) the effects of living in extremely poor or distressed neighbourhoods; (v) lack of access to good-quality services.

❑   Social exclusion presents a number of interlinked problems for social workers to deal with, in the form of individuals with depression and poor mental health, families under stress, children living in poverty, and older people cut off from activities and social engagement. Rather than self-standing problems they are intertwined with larger social conditions and stressors. Perhaps the biggest challenge for social workers in tackling social exclusion is to develop approaches that deal with these problems on a neighbourhood or community level.

KEY READING

Tom MacInnes and several others, *Monitoring Poverty and Social Exclusion 2014* (New Policy Institute and the Joseph Rowntree Foundation, 2014). The authors measure the extent of social exclusion in Britain based on a range of important indicators. The information is provided in clear graphs; produced annually.

John Hills, *Good Times Bad Times* (Policy Press, 2015). The chief researcher at the Centre for Analysis of Social Exclusion combines hard data with a reflective exploration of exclusion in an informative, very readable account.

Gerald Smale, Graham Tuson and Daphne Statham, *Social Work and Social Problems: Working Towards Social Inclusion and Social Change* (Macmillan, 2000). The late, far-seeing Gerry Smale and colleagues describe how in practice social workers can move from providing short-term aid to families to long-term development work and social change.

CHAPTER 2

SOCIAL WORK VALUES, POVERTY AND EXCLUSION

THIS CHAPTER COVERS

- Why values are important.

- Social work values and attitudes toward poverty inequality.

- The challenges to social work values from reform of the welfare system.

- The concept of social justice in a market society.

- Toward a new framework for social work values.

Social work is a distinctive profession because of the way it intertwines personal support and guidance to individuals and families with the quest for social justice. Each line of work is backed up by different sets of values, often with some tension between them. Despite their diversity of origins, with additions made over time, contemporary social work values to an extent have solidified and not responded to the fresh challenges and dilemmas that practitioners actually face. There is a danger of values remaining unchanged in a changing world.

This chapter aims to help practitioners make sense of values, particularly in relation to poverty and exclusion, and to enable them to examine their own value base in the face of specific moral challenges that they face.

WHAT ARE VALUES?

Expressed in codes of ethics, in social work degree programmes and in accumulation of moral preoccupations over decades, social work values represent the profound aspirations of professional commitment, 'held aloft as the ultimate and, perhaps, never wholly attainable ends of policy and practice', as Chris Clark has put it (Clark 2000: 31).

While values can be thought of as embedded in persons, professions and organisations, they are less precise than we might presume, pointing to, but not dictating, suggested courses of action. They are cumulative and build on each other to form an emerging tradition of commitments. As Clark says, they are 'the ongoing accomplishments of knowledgeable and reflective human intelligences immersed in a social world' (ibid.: 31).

Clark finds four broad principles present in social work values:

1   The worth and uniqueness of every person: all persons have equal value regardless of age, gender, ethnicity, physical or intellectual ability, income or social contribution. Respect for individuals is active and needs to be positively demonstrated rather than just assumed.
2   Entitlement to justice: every person is entitled to equal treatment on agreed principles of justice that recognise protection of liberties, human needs and fair distribution of resources.
3   Claim to freedom: every person and social group is entitled to their own beliefs and pursuits unless it restricts the freedom of others.
4   Community is essential: human life can only be realised interdependently in communities and much of social work aims to restore or improve specific communities.

(Clark 2000)

VALUES ARE NOT SET IN STONE

Social work values are more general and less directive than we might assume. As Clark writes:

> The evidence for the existence of a distinctive and coherent set of normative professional social work values is extremely tenuous; and the actual range and content of social workers' personal and professional values can be conjectured from the professional literature but is not evidenced by any significant body of empirical social research. The identification of social work values can therefore be no more than approximate, provisional and inherently controversial. In broad terms, the values of social work are clearly rooted in Christian ethics blended with modern Western secular liberal individualism. They share their origins with the dominant Western tradition of morality.

(Clark 2000: 360)

One of the most profound and difficult questions the profession faces concerns the nature of poverty and why some people are poor and some are not. Social work has worked with people in poverty since the origins of the profession in the second half of the nineteenth century. Yet to this day its values about poverty are contradictory and at times evasive. One thread, dating back to the origins of social work, was the 'pathologising' of poor people, that is, viewing users' poverty as the result of perverse choices – wilfully chosen addiction, irresponsible spending habits, apathetic attitude toward work and failing to recognise parental responsibilities. This deep-seated belief prompted social workers to focus on 'character', delve into household expenditure and offer guidance on users' moral conduct, and led to two of the earliest (and still potent if often disguised) assessment categories: the 'deserving' and the 'undeserving' poor (Pierson 2011).

The dominant casework tradition in social work built on this framework; its philosophical individualism deriving, as Clark noted above, from both a Christian and secular emphasis on individual uniqueness. It aimed to understand the user's life in his or her social environment and to achieve individual and family change with techniques such as counselling, and if needed with compulsory interventions sanctioned by law (Pearson 1989). The worker's relationship with that individual became central. A Catholic priest, Father Biestek (1961), codified these in the principles of casework that provided the foundation for the user–social work relationship:

- uniqueness of each individual
- purposeful expression of feelings
- controlled emotional involvement
- acceptance
- non-judgemental attitude
- client self-determination
- confidentiality.

From this perspective, poverty was too often seen as the inevitable backdrop to service provision and the responsibility of other agencies. Although criticised for putting too much emphasis on the individual relationship between client and practitioner and not enough on the social environments of users (Pearson 1989; Jones 2005), the principles of casework continue to influence how social workers view their work and in particular the remedies for tackling exclusion, despite evidence showing that users' poverty remains the single factor most widely associated with social work contact.

USERS ARE SMARTER THAN YOU THINK

Some users have long understood social workers' undying interest in depth psychology and family relationships as the platform from which they launch their work. Clients could sometimes work this to their advantage. 'Tailgunner' Parkinson, an old-school probation officer known for his capacity to pierce social work's pretensions, captured this four decades ago in a short article entitled simply 'I give them money'. He wrote, 'clients tried to talk about the gas bill, workers tried to talk about the client's mother. Perceptive clients got the gas bill paid by talking about their mother' (Parkinson 1970, cited in Dowling 1999).

SOCIAL WORK ATTITUDES TO POVERTY AND INEQUALITY

Overlaid on the casework emphasis on the individual were social democratic values associated with the post-war establishment of the welfare state in the late 1940s. Commitments in the 1960s to build preventive services to help families in poverty and to universalise social work services in comprehensive local authority departments moved on to include more explicit anti-poverty objectives. Radical social work in the 1970s sought to change economic and social structures, while somewhat later anti-oppressive practice from the 1980s on has sought to reverse major forms of discrimination based on 'race', masculinity, homophobia and Islamophobia (Pierson 2011). The notion of empowerment provided yet another set of commitments, enabling people without power to have more control over their lives and greater voice within institutions and extending a person's ability to take effective decisions (Braye and Preston-Shoot 1995: 48).

REFLECT AND DECIDE: WHAT ARE THE CAUSES OF POVERTY?

Reflect on the following questions: Are people poor because of personal failures and bad choices for which they bear responsibility? Does social work's commitment to equal opportunity mean that practice should directly tackle barriers that limit opportunity as a cause of poverty? Is the professional commitment to social justice too 'political'?

Various surveys have found ambivalence among social workers as to the causes of poverty throughout the profession (Bullock 2004; Craig 2001; Sun 2001; Garrett 2002). Gilligan for instance found that incoming social work students tend to think that poverty, along with other social problems, is the consequence of actions and behaviour of individuals, giving less attention to social or neighbourhood factors that may contribute to a family's low income. Over half the students he surveyed thought individual ignorance and failure of personal responsibility lay behind users' poverty. His study suggested that even those social work programmes adopting a strong emphasis on structural explanations would struggle to get their message across (Gilligan 2007: 739).

At the top end of the profession a similar ambivalence exists. Monnickendam and colleagues showed that directors of social services in Israel were unsure of their professional role and responsibilities in relation to users' poverty. They did not perceive the poor as a target for services and instinctively preferred intervention at individual and family level rather than tackling neighbourhood or social conditions that shaped users' poverty (Monnickendam et al. 2010).

The consequence of this ambivalence is that poverty is too often 'not seen' as a factor in users' lives. The burden that poverty places on individuals and families goes unrecognised and at the same time reinforces the conviction that poverty is a matter of personal individual responsibility, which fits more easily into the individualised value orientation that social work practice has long gravitated towards. Formal assessment

processes encourage this by excluding or minimising references to users' economic circumstances or neighbourhood environment. This is particularly the case in assessment
of children in need where matters such as low income and disadvantaged neighbourhood environments are often seen as simply givens about which little can be, or should
be, done. Practitioner ambivalence toward user poverty is reflected perhaps also in the
reluctance to take on advocacy roles or engage in local campaigns or pressure groups.

Codes of ethics: the call for social justice

Social work codes of ethics stipulate that social justice should be promoted through
advocacy work; presumably this includes tackling poverty and social exclusion although
neither of those terms appear in the codes.

REFLECT AND DECIDE: BRITISH ASSOCIATION OF SOCIAL WORK CODE OF ETHICS

The professional mandate for social workers includes a call for political advocacy on behalf
of social justice:

> The British Association of Social Workers puts it this way: 'Social workers have a
> duty to . . . bring to the attention of their employers, policy makers, politicians and
> the general public situations where resources are inadequate or where distribution of
> resources, policies and practice are oppressive, unfair, harmful or illegal'.
> (BASW 2012: Section 2.2)

How far does the code insist that practitioners explicitly tackle poverty and exclusion? What
does having a duty to 'bring to the attention of their employers . . . [and] politicians' mean
when faced with an unfair or oppressive allocation of resources? What form might this
take? What happens if the powers that be ignore the call?

It is evident that there is an ongoing struggle within the profession to meet its own
standards. Generally, the more formal the discourse (written documents such as codes
of ethics, mission statements, public professional reports), the more that discourse tends
to reflect the profession's declared statements on social justice. The more informal the
discourse (for example, intra-profession conversations, staff meetings, corridor talk),
the less focused it is on social justice. Jobs on offer, for example, rarely mention poverty
or recruiting persons to posts with specific roles tackling poverty. Krumer-Nevo and colleagues (2011) analysed seventy-five job descriptions to judge the extent to which they
were 'poverty aware', whether references to poverty appeared in defining users' situations
and whether goals and methods of intervention were mentioned to relieve poverty. They
found what they called a 'textual silence' in relation to poverty. The job descriptions,
they concluded, offered and simultaneously reproduced a conservative and apolitical
perspective on poverty and on social work practice with people living in poverty.

There are periodic calls for social workers to act more vigorously in accordance with stated codes to promote social justice. Davis and Wainright (2005), Craig (2002) and Mantle and Backwith (2010), among many others, urge social workers to adopt a 'poverty-aware' approach based on a detailed understanding of poverty's impacts on the lives of users, seeing poverty as a source of family distress, and the way it constrains choices in everyday life. Users' lack of material, social and symbolic resources should be targeted for intervention, just as other objectives are targeted, such as 'stopping spousal violence' or 'improving parental functioning'.

Beliefs about poverty

Professional values are only as effective as the practitioner makes them. For that reason personal values are extremely important too. Both professional and individual values may combine either to distance practitioners from or push them toward anti-poverty work. Personal beliefs about poverty are based in part on the practitioner's own upbringing and experiences and how familiar they are with what it is like to be poor, and in part on their understanding of society and what motivates individuals in conditions of scarcity. In the realm of values and beliefs it is easy to lose the complexity as to why a person, family or an entire neighbourhood is poor. Yet beliefs and values have a large influence on the way we understand explanations of poverty. For example, if you believe that people are themselves largely free to make choices for what happens to them in life, you quite likely will also think that people are poor because of personal failures for which they bear responsibility. Conversely, if you believe in equal opportunity for everyone, you may focus on the barriers that limit opportunity as a cause of poverty.

REFLECT AND DECIDE: UNDERSTANDING THE REALITY OF POVERTY

Here is a thought experiment. Imagine that you bank online and that you have responded to an email from the bank asking you to confirm your identity because there have been some suspicious withdrawals. The email asks for your user name and password – and, because you are very busy and preparing for a case conference in a couple of hours' time, you supply the information requested without reflection. An hour later your bank phones you to say that your account has been cleaned out and your debit card invalidated.

- What would your first reaction be?
- What would you actually do?
- Would you be able to concentrate on the conference as it went ahead?
- What would happen to the networking and relationship building with other professionals that you were planning on?

Now assume you are a lone parent with two small children, living on Job Seeker's Allowance paid into your bank account. You have just been informed that there is some official concern about your benefit that requires investigation and in the meantime benefit payments have been suspended, and you will be informed when they are to start again. Do you see similarities with the scenario above?

PHILOSOPHY OF WELFARE AND THE CHALLENGE OF WELFARE REFORM

In the nineteenth century, when such risks as injury, sickness or unemployment befell a person with no private means, they relied on family, received charity – or entered the workhouse where a subsistence living could be obtained. The classical welfare state, established after World War II, had a better idea: protect the individual and his (and it was largely 'his') dependants from adverse life events by pooling risk, creating in effect a nation-wide insurance system based on taxation. The aim was to guarantee a safety net for all, so that should a person fall out of the labour market (or fall sick, or be destitute in old age, or need care), that person would have a basic income and sufficient services to see them through. That safety net was not confined to income maintenance but extended to housing in the form of council housing (in a Britain that suffered massive destruction of property during World War II), to health in the form of the NHS, and to raising children in the form of family allowance. All paid in, all were supported when in need. In short, risks were collectively covered.

As important as the safety net was for individuals and for equality and social cohesion, the articulated philosophy of welfare was among the classical welfare state's greatest achievements. Particularly important in this philosophy was the notion of social rights to set alongside the legal and political rights established in earlier centuries. The work of T.H. Marshall (1950), Richard Titmuss (1966), Peter Townsend (1979), and others of international repute, established the right of all citizens including welfare claimants to participate fully in society and to share in the wellbeing of that society. The point of the welfare state, they argued, is to protect individuals and their families from becoming a mere commodity within the labour market. In extending this philosophy, in making it real in practice, social work was a willing participant, impatient with the limits of the welfare state at times and often advocating an extension of claimants' rights, but nevertheless fully signed up to this immense social democratic achievement.

While the classical welfare state has been under pressure for three decades, it faced a mortal threat in the years after 2010, its ethos shattered by the Great Recession and 'austerity' in government policy. For those who had grown up within the classical welfare state and defended its integrity and ethos throughout their lives, the experience has been traumatic. (See, for example, 'What happened to the world my generation built?' by Harry Leslie Smith, *Guardian*, 5 June 2014.) The new welfare system, instead of cushioning individuals and the family from the demands of the labour market when needed, seeks the opposite: a system that promotes the discipline of the labour market and ensures that all will submit to that discipline. This transition is clearest in relation to applicants for Universal Credit (UC) and disability claimants, where benefits are lost as punishment for not seeking work aggressively enough – but it is evident throughout the system, for example in relation to young people no longer eligible for any benefit, or single adults of working age.

'Risk shift'

The risks to income associated with unemployment, accident or sickness, with cognitive or physical disability or with mental health problems are no longer pooled and responded to collectively but are to be borne by the individual and family – what Jacob Hacker has called the 'great risk shift' (Hacker 2009). To get through life without major periods of financial hardship now requires a high degree of good luck, self-organisation and self-responsibility, but most of all, money. If a person has the money and the resources he or she may buy the services needed to support and protect themselves and their family – the kinds of support once offered by the classical welfare state. If a person does not have these resources she or he is forced to turn to the state-provided benefit system that is geared to getting the individual back to work as soon as possible. The benefit system has become a system of largely negative incentives to steer behaviour toward work readiness. Providing a service or benefit based on 'need' is replaced by a system that requires particular behaviours – job finding, job holding, job training.

Paradoxically the substantial rise in income inequality in the wake of the Great Recession – with huge gains in income and wealth for the top 1 per cent and stagnant wages for the working and middle class – has been a force in persuading parts of the public to acquiesce in cutting welfare benefits and tying benefits to work-related behaviour. This is not what one might have expected: news about increasing inequality appears to have made the public *less* trusting of government in general and less trusting in government to fix the problem of inequality in particular.

The sanctions system

Under rules for work-related benefits, sanctions are imposed on hundreds of thousands of people annually who, for whatever reason, do not or cannot comply with orders to find work, train for work or join the work programme as directed to do. Many more are under threat of sanctions. Understanding the sanction system – both from a practical and philosophical point of view – is an essential part of the social worker's knowledge base. It should drive advocacy on behalf of users since it contravenes basic human rights and the principles of procedural fairness. Those principles, grounded in concepts of natural justice, ensure that a fair and objective decision is reached on matters that vitally affect an individual's interests. They are there to protect the rights of individuals and to enhance public confidence in the decision-making process that could have severe and detrimental effect on individuals involved.

THE PRINCIPLES OF PROCEDURAL FAIRNESS

- *A fair hearing* – where certain interests and rights of an individual may be adversely affected by a decision maker, that person must be given details of the case against them and the opportunity to prepare and present evidence, after which the decision maker must respond to that evidence.
- *The bias rule* – the decision maker should be impartial, reaching a decision on a considered assessment of evidence before them; there should be no conflict of interest on the part of the decision maker.
- *The evidence rule* – the decision maker should be able to base their decision on specific evidence and not speculation.

The sanctioning process ignores all of these. Sanctions are in fact large financial penalties imposed on individuals by officials directly responsible to the Secretary of State who themselves are subject to pressures and performance targets unknown to the public at large (House of Commons 2014). Claimants are not present when decisions are made, nor do they have legal representation of any kind at any stage of decision making.* The scale of penalties that Universal Credit or Jobcentre Plus staff may impose is far higher than any magistrates court may impose for criminal misdemeanours, and unlike those of magistrates, the orders cannot be phased in to allow time for the claimant to re-adjust to paying the penalty but are effective immediately. Nor may penalties be varied because of impact on the individual or family – as magistrates are allowed to do with those convicted (Webster 2015). The introduction of 'mandatory reconsideration' of decisions in 2013, rather than a step toward fair hearing, is a further barrier to an appeal since it must happen before any appeal is lodged. Since there is no time limit for carrying out a mandatory reconsideration, claimants, including Employment Support Allowance claimants, may be without benefit for a lengthy period pending the outcome of the mandatory reconsideration.

Bias in decision making is institutionalised. For instance Schildrick and colleagues (2012: 67) examined the attitudes of welfare to work agency staff in Teesside. They found strong similarities between staff attitudes and those of employers taking part in work programme schemes. These favoured 'the right attitude, motivation and flexibility' in individual claimants above any qualifications or skills those claimants might have. In short, staff made subjective judgements on individual levels of motivation *over and above the skills claimants had already attained or stated they wanted to attain*. Schildrick *et al.* were surprised by this finding in light of the emphasis on acquiring skills in DWP policy.

Other, covert pressures came to light in this and other accounts of decision making on sanctions. There is some evidence to suggest, for instance, that targets are

*At the time of writing there has been limited judicial oversight of this process. One exception is the decision in R (Reilly and Wilson) v SSWP [2013] UKSC 68 at para 65 where the court held that 'fairness' requires a claimant to have 'such information about the [work] scheme as he or she may need in order to make informed and meaningful representations to the decision–maker before a decision is made' (cited in National Association of Welfare Rights Advisers 2014).

set in relation to the numbers of claimants to be sanctioned; in other words decisions are taken in advance that a certain percentage of claimants will be sanctioned regardless of individual circumstances, although this is disputed by the DWP. Nevertheless workers in Jobcentre Plus offices have reported that individual claimants are reallocated for reporting purposes so that profiles appear 'normal'; that is, each officer can be shown to have sanctioned the 'right' number of claimants, even when an individual officer's sanctioning of claimants may have been negligible (Thomas 2015).

Faced with high workloads, limited time and resources, and with agency targets to meet, staff adopted a rough and ready appraisal on whether an individual claimant was seriously seeking work. The researchers found for instance among the staff they interviewed a strong belief in a local culture of worklessness – in other words staff believed in an area-wide reluctance to find work which they then saw as a serious barrier to individual applicants wanting to succeed in the labour market. Anecdotes about a single individual were repeated to interviewers from different sources, suggesting that a single semi-mythical case stood in as 'empirical' evidence for a wider attitude among work programme staff that many claimants were simply not trying – giving credence to discredited 'underclass' conceptualisations (Schildrick *et al.* 2012: 74).

Social work values under pressure

The general shift of responsibility to the individual, when facing adversity with less and less help available from public authorities, has been compounded by the Coalition and Conservative governments altering the purpose, philosophy and rationale of the welfare state. It has changed from one thing into another. The concept of human need has been reconstructed on a narrow basis with the capacity to work at its core. They have redefined child poverty (see Chapter 4) and appropriated the foundational concepts of social justice and fairness in support of this. Above all, once the property of the extreme right wing,* the notion of the moral underclass has been installed at the heart of Department for Work and Pensions policy, equating receipt of welfare benefits with dependency and loss of the will to work. The regime seeks behavioural change in relation to work attitudes, and holds the individual uniquely responsible for the difficulties she or he may find themselves in, without regard to impairments or health needs, economic causes of unemployment or care responsibilities to others (Dwyer and Wright 2014).

'UNDERCLASS' THINKING

It turns out that the clichés about role models are true. Children grow up making sense of the world around them in terms of their own experience. Little boys don't naturally grow up to be responsible fathers and husbands. They don't naturally grow up knowing how to get up every morning at the same time and go to work . . . And most

---

*Charles Murray, the ultra-right commentator, made two forays into Britain in the 1990s to propagate his theory of the underclass; see Murray (1996).

> emphatically of all, little boys do not reach adolescence naturally wanting to refrain from sex, just as little girls don't become adolescents naturally wanting to refrain from having babies. That's why single-parenthood is a problem for communities, and that's why illegitimacy is the most worrisome aspect of single-parenthood.
>
> (Murray 1996: 31)

To achieve its ends, government has used a few key tools – expansion of the market in health and social care, cuts to welfare benefits, and compelling claimants to work in order to receive benefits. While it can be easily pointed out that some of these tools were deployed by previous governments, including the Labour administrations after 1997, it was the intensity of their use that characterised the behaviour of the Coalition after 2010 and the Conservative government after 2015 – an instance of quantitative change producing qualitative change.

REFLECT AND DECIDE: A NEWSPAPER REPORTS ON WELFARE REFORM

Britain's problem families are costing taxpayers a whopping £30 billion a year, it was claimed today.

The dysfunctional behaviour of half a million households in the country is resulting in a major drain on public resources, with the size of our 'underclass' four times larger than first thought.

Ministers have demanded an end to the 'it's not my fault' culture which has allowed up to 120,000 problem families to avoid taking responsibility for their own lives.

(Duell 2014)

What are the main features of the underclass family as described in this newspaper article?

The question is: how far should social work *as a profession* contest, obstruct, resist this ideological package? We take a brief further look at each of the major ideological factors below.

Benefit cuts

Prior to introducing its signature benefits system, Universal Credit, designed to replace tax credits, the Coalition had already significantly reduced welfare benefits in several areas and provided clues as to what UC aims to do. Those changes included:

- an increase in the number of hours people had to work to claim Working Tax Credit;
- a significant restriction on eligibility for the contribution-based Employment Support Allowance;
- an under-occupancy penalty in social housing – known alternatively as the 'bedroom tax' (by the left) or 'spare bedroom subsidy' (by the right);
- abolition of the Social Fund and introduction of local welfare assistance schemes to cover emergency payments.

The move from council tax benefit to council tax support and the introduction of local welfare assistance schemes – both run and funded by local authorities – was particularly problematic for social work users, in part because national eligibility criteria were replaced with a myriad of different local schemes, and in part because the funding available to local authorities to cover both was substantially less. With many other claims on their spending, local authorities cut their commitments to both schemes.

REFLECT AND DECIDE: WHAT IS THE PLACE OF CHARITY IN SOCIAL WORK'S VALUE SYSTEM?

One of the consequences of welfare reform is the sizeable increase in use of food banks by those on low incomes. Some councils use referrals to food banks as part of their welfare assistance schemes (Lambie-Mumford 2014).

> Food banks are charity; no one would want to call them centres for feeding the poor but that is what they are. In the time of eroding commitment to publicly provided welfare programmes, voluntary and private charity has become widespread, accompanied by a positive aura with enthusiastic volunteers and a message of saving grace.
>
> (Poppendieck 1999: 7)

What value judgement should social work develop in relation to charity – and to food banks in particular? How far should social work 'own' the consequences of the expanding role of charity and the corresponding shrinking of state provision? When a charity collapses through insufficient funding, what should social work's public comment be?

REFLECT AND DECIDE: THE ROLE OF FOOD BANKS

Should referrals to food banks be seen as a normal, valid element within support services for impoverished families? One radical social work strategy is to meet need from charitable sources if no other is available, so long as a debate is initiated with service users as to the limits of charity and how they might become involved in advocating a rights-based provision. Is this a plausible strategy in your view?

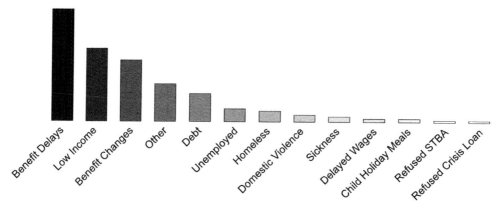

FIGURE 2.1   Reasons for referral to food banks, 2013–14 (Trussell Trust 2014; reproduced with permission from the Trussell Trust)

Specific households were hit particularly hard under the new welfare regime. For example some 444,000 people lost nearly £17 each week through the under-occupancy penalty (bedroom tax) (MacInnes *et al.* 2014). As a result of the first benefit cap at £25,000, 40,000 families lost an estimated £93 a week on average. As MacInnes *et al.* write: 'To lose a sum of money this large must require a drastic change in the way a family lives.' They argue that the incomes derived from the main means-tested benefits were already low, worth 60 per cent of the Minimum Income Standard for families with children and just 40 per cent for single working-age adults – with the latter only just able to cover what the public thinks is necessary for a minimum living standard: food, fuel and water (ibid.).

FROM COUNCIL TAX BENEFIT TO COUNCIL TAX SUPPORT

The introduction of council tax support (CTS) meant that 326 local schemes across England replaced a single central system – with 10 per cent less funding in total than the old council tax benefit. Moreover, whereas the previous system guaranteed 100 per cent cover for claimants' council tax, initially only forty-five of the local schemes maintained that level of complete support. Nor did that small number last long. For local authorities, who cannot increase council tax in general by more than 2 per cent without holding a referendum, cutting CTS entitlement is a way of increasing revenue – presenting low-income families with higher council tax payments year on year (Bushe *et al.* 2014).

Markets

Those who justify markets as the pre-eminent means by which to allocate goods and services argue, first, that they underpin freedom and individual liberty because all can participate according to their preferences, and second, markets have the unrivalled capacity to process information on supply and demand of goods and services. They crunch an infinity of consumer purchases and organise as efficiently as possible the production of products or services and the price for those products or services. No centrally planned economy could undertake that work as efficiently, so the argument goes.

REFLECT AND DECIDE: THE ROLE OF MARKETS

Markets require individuals to buy care on the social care market. What does a well-ordered care market look like? As the cost of care rises, how does this affect our feelings about care? Why are care workers paid so little for providing hands-on social care? Should social work's code of ethics commit itself to minimising the extent of markets in social care provision? In family support services for children and families?

Pro-market arguments rest on the belief that markets are inherently virtuous and should be allowed to determine the allocation of goods and services in all areas of civil and social life, while all government attempts to regulate them should be eliminated. Hand in hand with belief in the superiority of markets comes belief in a small state – sometimes referred to as the 'night watchman' state since all it should do is keep the peace. Some of the most impassioned defenders of the market mechanism are libertarians who favour unfettered markets and oppose government regulation not in the name of economic efficiency but in the name of human freedom.

FREE MARKET LIBERTARIANS ARGUE THAT . . .

. . . inherent in freedom is the right to do what one wants with the things that one owns, provided we respect that freedom for others. Many of the activities of the state, from this perspective, are illegitimate because they violate liberty. Opposition to the minimum wage is on the same basis. Charitable donation is the result of individual choice and thus accords with libertarian principles. Libertarians are opposed to all efforts to redistribute wealth or income – or indeed any law that compels some people to help others, including governments raising taxes to provide financial assistance to those in need. The minimal state exists only to enforce contracts, keep the peace and protect private property. Taxing the rich to help the poor coerces the rich. The principle of self-ownership is central – I own myself, I own my labour and am entitled to the fruits of that labour. To tax the return I get on my labour is to take hours of my life from me. Taxation = forced labour = slavery.

(adapted from Robert Nozick's *Anarchy, State and Utopia*, 1974)

REFLECT AND DECIDE: REGULATING PENSIONERS' SPENDING

One of the leading exponents of free markets, Milton Friedman, said this in 1962: 'If a man knowingly prefers to live for today, to use his resources for current enjoyment, deliberately choosing a penurious old age, by what right do we prevent him from doing so?' (Friedman 1962: 188).

Referring to the new freedom to withdraw money from individual pension accounts, Steve Webb, Minister for Pensions, said this in 2014: 'So actually, if people do get a Lamborghini, and end up on the state pension, the state is much less concerned about that, and that is their choice' (*Guardian*, 20 March 2014).

Should pensioners be free to spend their accumulated pension in one go?

Austerity

Coalition and subsequent Conservative government policy has been the most important agent in undermining the classical welfare state ethos and replacing it with something quite opposite. Since 2010, 'austerity' and the political arguments in its favour have persuaded the public that only deep cuts in public expenditure will ensure the return of prosperity by creating confidence for the private sector. The Coalition articulated a moral dimension to austerity suggesting shared sacrifice. 'Austere' in everyday parlance means simple, strict, severe, suggesting that while the sacrifices are tough, they are a much-needed antidote to years of government overspend. Quite apart from the fact that managing the budget of a country is not remotely similar to managing that of a single household (see Krugman 2013), this hides the fact that government, under the mask of austerity, chose specific targets to be 'austere' with. 'Austerity' has in fact meant specific reductions resulting in specific losses to specific people. Pensions for older people have not suffered, for example, whereas benefits for young people and funding for youth services have been drastically cut. For people who do not use any of the affected services, these cuts have no downside. For those who rely on local authority services, the consequences are enormous, especially in the most disadvantaged authorities where the cuts have fallen the hardest (Krugman 2015; see also Blyth 2014).

REFLECT AND DECIDE: DOES SOCIAL WORK'S CODE OF ETHICS NEED TO BE CHANGED?

Does social work's code of ethics (see above) need to be changed to respond explicitly to the role that markets in social care now play in its provision? Does austerity have a moral dimension that needs to be addressed – either in support or contesting – by social work ethical codes? Should social workers' code of ethics say anything regarding benefit cuts and what social workers should do in relation to users who have had their benefits cut?

SOCIAL JUSTICE, SOCIAL RIGHTS AND SOCIAL WORK

Social work values at the very least need to respond more explicitly to the challenges outlined above: to think through where it stands as a profession on a variety of matters – sanctions, the place of the market, how far advocacy should become a major part of practice. One way to begin this work is to consider again what the foundation values of social work are in the twenty-first century.

For example, the commitment to social justice finds its way into virtually all social work codes of ethics across the globe, including Britain. Of course no one argues against the concept of social justice, or in favour of social injustice. But what does it actually mean? For much of its history the concept was rooted in a discourse of human rights and social rights found widely in United Nations declarations. The concept has been richly articulated by some of the best theorists of the classical welfare state. As T.H. Marshall put it, the state has certain social responsibilities towards its citizens, moving from providing 'the right to a modicum of economic welfare and security to the right to share to the full in the social heritage and to live the life of a civilized being according to the standards prevailing in the society' (Marshall 1950). He wrote:

> Components of a civilized and cultured life, formerly the monopoly of the few, were brought progressively within reach of the many, who were encouraged thereby to stretch out their hands toward those that still eluded their grasp. The diminution of inequality strengthened the demand for its abolition, at least with regard to the essentials of social welfare.
>
> (Marshall 1950: 47)

The welfare state was not confined to allowing 'the most vulnerable among us' to eke out a life on benefits, but offered collective provision, universalistic in its ambition, sufficient to ensure that all would thrive.

But the concept of social justice is now heavily contested following the Coalition's adoption of the term for its own purposes,* which raises the questions: (a) what does it *actually* entail; and (b) by what means can it be delivered? The White Paper on tackling poverty took social justice in a completely different direction: '[It] is about making society function better – providing the support and tools to help turn lives around' (HM Government 2012). The White Paper provides no definition of social justice – rather it is summed up as a collection of social phenomena:

- Measuring poverty by income alone is not the way to measure poverty.
- Providing income support to poor families is not the way to bring people out of poverty: 'Income through benefits maintains people on a low income, and can even risk bolstering welfare dependency and feeding social problems such as drug dependency'.
- Preserving family stability is first and foremost the way society leaves poverty behind. Families are not helped by focusing on income.
- Social justice is realised by tackling worklessness within households, supporting two-parent families and underpinning the stability of parental relationships,

*This was foreshadowed when the former leader of the Conservative Party, Iain Duncan Smith, set up the Institute of Social Justice in 2001.

reducing the size of the gap in educational attainment between children from low-income families and their peers, and reducing drug dependency, debt and crime.

The structural forces that impinge on family life, the focus of much public effort of social work institutions and practitioners – racism, disability, sexism, material deprivation – are dismissed in this short paragraph:

> We know that in *some cases* these disadvantages can be exacerbated by factors like ethnicity, gender or disability. For instance, disabled people are substantially more likely to experience material deprivation than people who are not disabled. *This strategy does not focus on these factors as themes* – rather it looks at the areas of disadvantage and how best to tackle them. This is not to ignore the role that factors like these can play in contributing to multiple disadvantages, however, and the importance of changing that picture.
>
> (my italics; HM Government 2012)

What the White Paper is saying is that widespread disadvantage (it does not use the phrase social exclusion but clearly has it in mind) is caused by certain behaviours, especially family breakdown, separation and divorce, which it returns to again and again. Gender and disability may exacerbate this disadvantage *but the primary cause is the divorce rate, addiction and failure to track the progress of adolescents.* Social justice is achieved by getting people to change their behaviour – for example by not getting divorced. Providing income support for poor families is not part of social justice: the cuts to welfare offered by the Conservative Party in the wake of the 2015 general election are based precisely on this logic.

This discourse represents a serious challenge to social work's long assumption, enshrined in its codes of ethics, that it unproblematically embodies practice toward a progressively fairer society. The challenge comes from the top of government with the force of statute behind it, a discourse that aims specifically at removing from social work its role of advocating for a more just society. The government has challenged social work on its own territory, so to speak, demanding it change its vision and commitments. Three moments particularly underscored this: (i) the proposal to put child safeguarding out to market (subsequently withdrawn under the Coalition); (ii) putting probation work out to tender by private suppliers; and (iii) the Secretary of State for Education's declaration that social work should not concern itself with social justice (Gove 2013).

Basic argument for social justice: fairness

In the face of this challenge, a profession-wide discussion is required to revisit the value base and to think anew social work's commitments. Fairness in society is a starting point, making it clearer what social work means by social justice.

John Rawls (1971) argues that justice is fairness. In a powerful thought experiment Rawls asks us to imagine we are rational individuals who wish to build a fair and just society but that none of us knows what social positions, abilities, hardships, income levels, or aspirations we will experience in life. We have no idea whether we will be in the top tenth of income or the bottom tenth, no idea what our individual strengths would be or the social circumstances we would find ourselves in. Nor have we any idea whether we will be intelligent or skilful enough in life to succeed and triumph over adversity. This he calls 'the veil of ignorance' – not knowing anything about where we will end up in life or what kind of welfare system (if any) society will construct for those who fall on hard times.

This position of ignorance, Rawls argues, compels us to think about what is universally fair. Since we have no idea where we will end up in terms of social or economic advantage (and could just as easily be among the bottom tenth as the top tenth), we are inescapably led to settle on two principles of justice:

1   The guarantee of equal basic rights and liberties sufficient to secure the fundamental interests of all including a wide variety of conceptions of a meaningful life.
2   Ensuring equal educational and employment opportunities as well as – and this is critical to his concept of justice – a guaranteed minimum of means, including income and wealth for all so that they could pursue their interests and maintain their self-respect as free and equal persons. Rawls does make room for inequality in his philosophy *as long as* the least advantaged in some way benefit by that inequality (Rawls 1971).

REFLECT AND DECIDE: THE VEIL OF IGNORANCE

Place yourself behind the veil of ignorance. Assuming then that you know nothing about your circumstances, abilities and how your life will turn out – what principles of fairness would you wish to see at the heart of society? Would you want to see a meaningful life guaranteed for all, a life of self-respect open to all regardless of behaviour, or would you put some qualifications on that? Do you think that inequality of income and wealth, for example, is justified as a reward for those who start productive businesses or make important scientific findings? What kind of welfare system would you sketch out? Do you think Rawls's notion of a guaranteed 'minimum of means' including income is justified? Do you think those currently enjoying high levels of wealth are truly able to engage with this thought experiment?

Should there then be enforced equality across the board? Rawls says no. He promotes what he calls 'the difference principle' – everyone should be encouraged to develop their abilities and capacities to the full but with the understanding that the rewards that they obtain in the market place belong to the community as a whole. The strongest runners should not be held back; however they should 'acknowledge in advance that the winnings don't belong to them alone, but should be shared with those who lack similar gifts' (Sandel 2009: 156).

A HYPOTHETICAL STATEMENT OF VALUES IN RELATION TO MARKETS

Caring for people is a social obligation that extends beyond the commercial realm. Although ownership of social care delivery may also rest in private companies, care itself cannot be owned and must be viewed as a service that is rendered and remunerated under the stewardship of those in the health and social care system rather than merely sold to individuals or communities. The social and health care of individuals and families is at the centre of delivery but must be practised within the overall context of continuing work to generate the greatest possible gains in wellbeing for whole communities.

In theory Britain is a 'meritocratic market society' – everyone finds their place according to their skills and abilities. In theory all may enter the race to success – but there are different starting points, with some much closer to the finishing line while others are blocked at the start.* In this sense, meritocracy confers hidden and unfair advantages that are both physical and intellectual but also class- and wealth-based: social connections, internships passed out within elite networks, heavy emphasis on communicative skills early in life, income sufficient to afford university tuition; meanwhile other families have to draw on charity – in the form of food banks – to survive.

Social workers engage largely with those in the bottom income quartile, and it is those on the lowest income who suffer directly from exclusionary inequality that should be the focus of fairness according to justice principles. Regarding inequality, public attitudes as well as political thinking regularly dismiss the solution that was for decades at the heart of addressing inequality: redistribution of income. And perhaps because of this drift away from remedies based on redistribution, inequality does not loom large in social work's values either.

But the extreme inequality of contemporary Britain should matter to social workers and to social work. In a highly unequal Britain, a wealthy stratum, able to protect and insure itself against risks, opposes those in poverty who cannot so protect themselves, who live day by day, dealing with an implacable scarcity, a pressure that cannot be relieved, 'the deadline that never lifts'.

All professional decisions are moral. Ethics is the capacity to think critically about moral values and direct our actions in terms of those values. There are different ways to express these values, and social work, a veritable laboratory for examining the effects of poverty, needs to think deeply on such questions.

---

*The French author, Anatole France, put it this way: 'The law, in its majestic equality, forbids the rich as well as the poor to sleep under bridges, to beg in the streets, and to steal bread'.

KEY POINTS

❏   Social workers have long been ambivalent in their values and attitudes toward poverty and social exclusion.

❏   Social work's casework tradition and commitment to social justice are intertwined, but face challenges from welfare reform and the re-emergence of the concept of the underclass in government policy.

❏   Sanctioning welfare claimants presents a particular challenge to social work's values as the process ignores every element of natural justice.

❏   Social workers have long been familiar with the effects of social exclusion on individuals and families – family breakdown, mental and physical ill health, educational under-achievement, unemployment and loss of self-esteem; they are in a better position than others to negotiate the complex boundaries between individual and social dynamics to achieve a greater measure of that social justice, but need to think through the specific nature of that commitment.

KEY READING

Daniel Dorling, *Injustice: Why Social Inequality Persists* (Policy Press, 2009). This socially conscious geographer graphically outlines the nature of inequality.

Chris Clark, *Social Work Ethics: Politics, Principles and Practice* (Macmillan, 2000). Clark stresses the contingent, evolving nature of values rather than as fixed dogma.

Gary Craig, Tania Burchardt and David Gordon, *Social Justice and Public Policy Seeking Fairness in Diverse Societies* (Policy Press, 2008). The authors provide a good overview of the issues as well as a discussion on John Rawls and other philosophers of justice.

CHAPTER 3

TACKLING EXCLUSION IN PRACTICE

THIS CHAPTER COVERS

- Five building blocks for tackling social exclusion in practice.

- The basics of the new welfare system.

- Social work roles and responsibilities to promote inclusion.

- Evidence base for a practice promoting inclusion and fairness.

The chapter introduces five building blocks for working with socially excluded individuals, groups and neighbourhoods. The building blocks are generic – they apply to social work with all groups of users. Some may be familiar, others will be new, prompting the need to think about roles and responsibilities. The first – securing a basic income for users – is dealt with at greater length because of the revolution in welfare benefits introduced by the Coalition and Conservative governments from 2010 on. The others have emerged from the changed landscape within which social workers now work – smaller state and larger markets – or from research about how the process of social exclusion works. In brief, they ask the practitioner to be flexible, neighbourhood-focused and willing to collaborate with other services. This ensemble of practice approaches, and the knowledge base behind it, fills out the link been social work and a just society.

The five building blocks are:

- Securing a basic income and basic resources for users and their families.
- Strengthening social supports and networks.
- Working in partnership with agencies and local organisations.

- Creating channels of effective participation for users, local residents and their organisations.
- Focusing on neighbourhood and community-level practice.

SECURING BASIC INCOME

Social workers are in the vital position of being able to assist users in examining the various means to improve their income levels. This inevitably takes both user and social worker into the complexities of the welfare system, work capability assessment and the precarious process through which claims are made and user needs met. Understanding the nature of the overhaul of welfare since 2010 is a critical first step to becoming an advocate on welfare matters.

Universal Credit

The prolonged, disorganised shift to Universal Credit (UC) means that the existing system of benefits, particularly working tax credits, will run side by side with the introduction of UC across the country over a period of several years. When and if UC is fully introduced the level of in-work supports, particularly for lone mothers, will be substantially less than under the current system of working tax credits. Overall, UC is a system for cutting benefits including the basic safety net benefits on which the welfare state has long been founded (Institute of Fiscal Studies 2014). UC is intended to be simpler and more cost effective than the previous benefits system and is best understood as a repackaging of previous benefits, with the rules for eligibility broadly carried over from the benefits it replaces. Its aim is to unify and simplify a range of older benefits, each with its own claiming process – an aim that is undermined through the many delays and lack of transparency that has hampered the scheme from the start.

Both UC and existing benefits such as Jobseekers Allowance and Employment and Support Allowance use incentives to move from benefits to work and, once in work, to increase hours worked. They aim to achieve this by reducing the rate at which benefits are withdrawn from those who find work and by adjusting the marginal tax rates faced by people moving from benefits to work, so that the individual retains more of their earnings. The housing costs element of UC, when it is introduced, will replace Housing Benefit and be paid directly to tenants in the social rented sector rather than to landlords, with some exceptions.

Sanctions and benefits

The welfare benefits system places heavy behavioural demands on claimants. Claimants' tax and pay information as well as job-searching activity are continually surveyed – with a suite of penalties at the discretion of job centre staff. Workless claimants are required to spend thirty-five hours a week seeking more or better-paid work. The 'part workless' are not exempt: experimental trials on the effects of interviews on claimant behaviour are under way, with one trial group having to submit to challenging interviews aiming to increase the claimant's hours worked and to reduce 'dependency' on the state.

The system has implications for mothers that are obvious but remain undiscussed. It will keep lone and low-paid mothers away from their children for unprecedented amounts of time. Single parents with children over 1 year old must attend 'work-focused interviews' or face sanctions; when a child turns 13 the parent is expected to obtain full-time work (including a maximum commute of ninety minutes); thus 13-year-olds face spending each day without their only carer (HM Government 2013). As Ruth Cain, a lecturer in law, has written: 'We can connect the extension of neoliberal "responsibilisation" rhetoric to low-paid "hardworking families" to the neoliberal assumption of total private responsibility for children – expressed in such truisms as "if you cannot afford children then don't have them"' (Cain 2015).

CASE STUDY: MS W

Ms W's 13-year-old son regularly bunks off school and she is already the subject of a parenting order stipulating that she get her child to school on time every day. Out of her wages she can just meet the costs of before- and after-school child care that starts at 7.30 am, when she begins her long commute to work, and finishes at 6 pm. When her son truants who will be held responsible? What are Ms W's options?

In relation to JSA, the Coalition government in October 2012 increased the minimum sanctioning period to four weeks for minor non-compliance, such as missing a meeting with an employment adviser, and to thirteen weeks for intermediate-level non-compliance, such as failing to apply for a job recommended by an adviser or failing to work without pay for privately contracted agencies. (In Chapter 2 we discussed how this process undermines principles of natural justice.)

The great majority of sanctions – 'adverse decisions' in DWP language – are imposed for claimants' failure to meet Jobcentre Plus requirements to make themselves available for work or work-related appointments. The numbers grew larger after the Coalition introduced a more demanding regime in October 2012 that applied sanctions to disabled persons and lone parents, making it among the harshest in Europe (Loopstra *et al.* 2015). The total number of people who received a sanction in one form or another, or were under threat of sanction, was close to 2 million for 2013, based on DWP figures. Of these, 120,000 claimants were classified as disabled. The total number of adverse decisions from across Great Britain was 1,444,411 (DWP 2014).

Whether sanctions work and actually encourage or pressure claimants into finding work is hotly contested. Defenders say that sanctions are a form of 'tough love' necessary to break an individual's or family's long-term reliance on welfare benefits. As Neil Couling, DWP work services director, told the Scottish Parliament's select committee, 'Some people no doubt react very badly to being sanctioned – we see some very strong reactions – but others recognise that it is the wake-up call that they needed, and it helps them get back into work' (Wintour 2014).

Other studies, however, have shown that sanctioned individuals end up more *disconnected* from work and from the welfare system. They have lower human capital – skills, training and education – and other disadvantages that suggest they would face barriers to complying with the extensive conditions for receiving unemployment benefits and have intentionally removed themselves from the system. There is a high correlation between the introduction of harsher sanctions and the substantial increase in persons leaving the system; they are not going into employment but to destinations unrelated to work. Loopstra and colleagues think there are several reasons for this: frequent interview requirements and the required hours of job search activity make it difficult for those with restricted access to transportation or a computer and mobile phone, and particularly those with young children, to meet requirements. Also processes for evaluating the needs of claimants and assessment of work capability are inadequate, potentially resulting in inappropriate placements. Finally it may be that claimants simply find the system dehumanising and stigmatising (Loopstra *et al.* 2015).

Supporting and advising a claimant

Social workers with families or individuals applying for working tax credits, JSA, ESA or UC when it is introduced, need to do three things. They should, first, be able to look across the benefits system to identify linked entitlements and the crossover possibilities within the system. Second, they need to be in a position to either directly help users negotiate the claiming process or be able to refer to the best sources of advice as to whether claimants would be better off or worse off following a particular claim on benefits. Income based Universal Credit, as with the current benefits system, will be a passport to other supports such as help with housing costs. This becomes critical when a user is facing sanctions and loss of income. Old dilemmas around balancing work and child care are only intensified in the new system. For example, if a mother increases her work to sixteen or more hours a week on average and has child-care responsibilities, she will continue to be eligible for tapered support through working tax credits or UC. This in turn raises difficult issues – what support does a young mother need in arranging care for her young children? Where is she to find the right care for her child? How is she to pay for it? Intangible matters also come into play – such as the social contacts outside the home that a job might bring weighed against the strain of juggling work and family.

Third, social workers should be able to offer sustained support throughout the claiming process. Claiming benefits is designed to provoke anxiety – the nature and demands of the process are themselves a deterrent to claiming benefit. Applications can only be completed and submitted digitally; there is no paper claim form, only limited telephone contact, and minimal face-to-face contact, if any. This is alien terrain for those not used to making online applications of any kind, let alone a matter of survival as this is. For those with literacy or language difficulties, with problems in picking up social and verbal cues, or with visual impairments or dyslexia, the claiming process becomes extremely difficult.

Young people are more affected by the rapid growth in benefit sanctions than any other age group. As Figure 3.1 indicates, the number of sanctions increased for all age groups but did so most for those under 25, with individuals in this group accounting for 41 per cent of all sanctions issued under the new regime from October 2012 to December 2013 (Watts 2014).

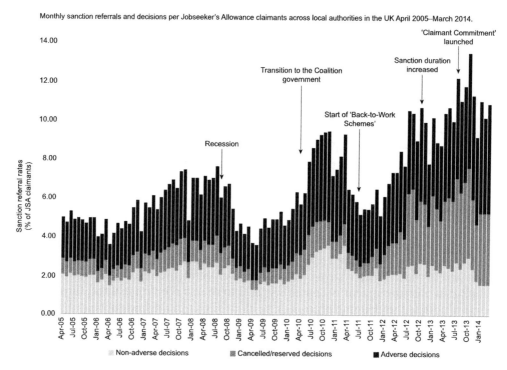

Monthly sanction referrals and decisions per Jobseeker's Allowance claimants across local authorities in the UK April 2005–March 2014.

FIGURE 3.1   Growth in the number of benefit sanctions (from Loopstra et al. 2015; reproduced with permission from the author)

CASE STUDY: MS C

Ms C, 46, has ME, severe depression and other health problems. She waited thirteen months – from September 2013 to October 2014 – to have her eligibility assessed for her Personal Independence Payment (PIP). In that year she could spend £8 per week on food that she bought from a local supermarket. That venture, once a week, was the only time she left her house. She had to travel some way to attend her face-to-face PIP assessment in spite of having told assessors that she found travelling difficult. She was told in that case her application would be cancelled. PIP assessment standards state that claimants must be willing to travel ninety minutes each way by public transport to an assessment centre.

Take-up campaigns

Benefit take-up campaigns in which communities and neighbourhoods are made aware of benefits that may be available to claimants are part of the approach to securing a minimum standard for all claimants. A significant proportion of eligible people do not claim the means-tested benefits to which they are entitled, whether unwilling to do so or through lack of information. In 2010 the total amount of unclaimed benefit was some £10 billion, with eligible working families responsible for nearly a third of that amount (Finn and Goodship 2014). In 2011–12 HMRC estimated that £3.29 billion in Working Tax Credit and 1.19 billion in Child Tax Credits went unclaimed (HMRC 2013). Improving the take-up of means-tested benefits and tax credits across the board contributes to poverty reduction – with associated improvements in health, family well-being and job retention – for the families social workers work with. Take-up campaigns combine a number of approaches:

- Initiatives at local level by local councils or advice services are particularly effective and typically generate more additional benefit income for low-income households than they cost.
- Simplifying the language and content of the application process, particularly regarding the verification of users' circumstances.
- Telephone and online applications – these can assist but also deter; users need direct coaching particularly for online applications.
- Using systematic feedback from users, front-line staff and advocates need to highlight problem areas in the system, especially where different multiple entitlements interact.
- Ensuring people are informed of entitlements at key points when they become eligible such as when registering a birth or receiving a medical diagnosis.
- Targeting take-up campaigns at hard-to-reach groups for benefits of small sums rather than high-value entitlements.
- Taking information into communities through outreach activities in partnership with trusted intermediaries such as health and community-based organisations.

(Finn and Goodship 2014: 8)

WHAT DOES THE TEAM KNOW ABOUT UNIVERSAL CREDIT?

At a team meeting, run through this checklist on the state of current preparation for securing basic resources for users under UC.

- Does your team – and do you individually – focus on the income of users and consider with them at regular intervals options as to how they might increase their income?
- Have you forged partnerships with other providers of expert advice such as social landlords, welfare to work agencies, charities and voluntary organisations, local support services for introducing Universal Credit, and health organisations involved with work capability assessments?
- Do you have a designated person responsible for keeping up to date with benefit rules?
- If you are in a local authority team is your department's charging policy for social care explained clearly and within the context of receipt of other benefits?
- Do you consider yourself well informed on the range of benefits that users might claim?
- Does your organisation have an anti-poverty strategy? Has it joined with other agencies to create a benefits take-up campaign?

Advocacy and the benefits system

Practitioners should prepare to act as advocates to achieve some semblance of fairness in the system, particularly in regard to work capability assessments (see Chapter 6). Faults and errors in the system are manifold – hidden targets, human error, misconduct and provocation, arbitrariness, hidden discrimination, flouting of rules and regulations by administrators, even missed telephone calls all occur but go undocumented (House of Commons 2014). Any of the following happen with some regularity:

- A claimant's failure to meet conditions because he or she fails to understand what is expected of them.
- Poor communication between Work Programme providers and Jobcentre Plus or UC staff leads to claimants being sanctioned though they have complied with requirements.
- The phenomenon of 'mass prescription' through which all claimants are given blanket instructions, regardless of circumstance and with no information about their sanctions (see case study below).
- A lower-level sanction is imposed *after* the claimant has re-engaged with his or her work requirements because the claimant does not understand what is required of them in terms of re-engagement. In such instances sanctions may run on for weeks or months (NAWRA 2014).
- An unfair decision arising from a conflict between disability and work requirements attached to a benefit claim.
- Issues of literacy, digital literacy, comprehension and level of education are shot through the whole process, and the social worker involved with a claimant has some responsibility to ensure that these needs are responded to.

There are then a number of questions for practitioners and users jointly to follow through on: do sanctioned claimants know why they have been sanctioned and, if not, can this be made clearer to them? Do claimants feel informed about the sanctions process? If not, how could they be better informed? Are claimants aware of sources of support and help available to them, including from Jobcentre Plus itself? Do they know how to appeal a decision to be sanctioned? In particular, when a sanction is imposed, the practitioner should know, if the clamant does not, how to apply for hardship payments through local welfare assistance schemes.

CASE STUDY: J

Claimant J is 18 years old with learning difficulties, and a care leaver. He claimed JSA as he wants to work, but asked to see the Disability Employment Adviser (DEA) because of his particular needs. However, due to long waiting times to get an appointment with the DEA, an appointment for the Work Programme was arranged first. The claimant did not understand the terms of the appointment, needed support that he did not receive and failed to attend. He was sanctioned but no written notification was sent and no opportunity for him to explain his non-attendance was offered. Nor were his particular needs taken into account even though he had specifically requested to see a DEA. The claimant only found out about the sanction when his benefit stopped (NAWRA 2014).

Two kinds of advocacy are relevant to shoring up fair treatment of claimants who are sanctioned or are otherwise refused a claim: individual case advocacy, in which work is focused on individuals or families, and systemic or 'cause' advocacy, where knowledge from individual cases contributes to a collective push for systemic change to legislation, policy and practice (Dalrymple and Boylan 2013: 3). For individual case advocacy, Neil Bateman (2005) has laid down six principles for effective advocacy:

1   Always act in the user's best interests. This principle is easily overlooked when facing multiple and competing pressures from managers in your own organisation or other agencies. It means constantly reminding yourself of the person on whose behalf you are acting.
2   Always act in accordance with the user's wishes and instructions; the advocate's actions have to be driven by these. Developing what Bateman calls an 'instructional relationship' is an important first step. Within this the advocate can identify facts, options and remedies, but will listen for the user's instructions.
3   Keep the user properly informed. She or he must know all essential facts related to their situation without being overwhelmed by information. Equally the user must be kept informed of all actions taken on their behalf. Accountability is impossible otherwise.
4   Carry out instructions with diligence and competence. If you offer to do something, make sure you do it – but know your limits and do not undertake that for which you are not prepared or competent.
5   Act impartially and offer frank, independent advice. This means being able to say uncomfortable things to representatives from other organisations (or your own) and not being beholden to the other side. A cooperative relationship based on partnership with the other side is not appropriate and can lead to a breach of advocacy principles.
6   Maintain the rules of confidentiality. Users must feel completely secure in the knowledge that what they say remains confidential.

(Bateman 2005)

BUILDING SOCIAL NETWORKS

A social network is the web of relationships through which people are connected. A network may be supportive or destructive, plentiful or virtually non-existent, close and intense or far-flung and distant. 'Network poverty' deprives users of social supports and informal help that we all need to participate in community life and to enjoy the standards of living shared by the majority of people.

Understanding the function of social networks and approaches to strengthening them when possible is an important element in overcoming the isolation of users. Our understanding both of the importance of social networks and how they function has developed considerably in the last twenty years. There are various ways of describing and measuring the characteristics of networks. One helpful distinction is to think of networks for 'getting by' and those for 'getting ahead'; they are very different and perform very different functions.

Networks for getting by

These are the close, supportive networks embedded in everyday relationships of friends, neighbourhood and family. When we think of the social supports offered by extended families and friends or by close-knit communities, these are networks for 'getting by'. Through these, last-minute gaps in child care are filled, a sick person is looked after, a small loan or cash to make ends meet is provided, and family celebrations or rites of passage are extended by their participation.

Social workers have a large investment in how these networks are viewed by the people with whom they are working. They may be seen as affirmative, nurturing and accepting or as antagonistic and inaccessible. At their very worst they can be sources of heavy responsibility, aggression and scapegoating. Understanding how such networks function helps us to understand better the distinctive characteristics of socially excluded and isolated individuals and families (Briggs 1997).

Networks for getting ahead

These networks provide crucial information for individuals and families on jobs, education, training and a range of options for advancing individual interests. In many ways they are the opposite of networks for getting by, but they can achieve important goals in their own right. Mark Granovetter has summed up this kind of network in the phrase 'the strength of weak ties' (Granovetter 1973). The 'weak ties' he refers to are the networks found outside the immediate neighbourhood and family and friends; they are occasional and episodic in nature and are more tenuous than a close personal relationship. They may be based on 'someone who knows someone' about a job possibility, or on the links obtained through a skills agency half a city away which a person visits only occasionally (Briggs 1997). Such networks are often referred to as 'bridging social capital' – the kind of network that provides access to institutions and employment markets that personal relationships simply cannot offer.

'Weak ties' can in fact be very powerful by providing information and opportunities for self-development. This is particularly so in relation to the jobs market, which has become complex and difficult to navigate for all young people, but particularly so for those from low-income urban neighbourhoods or adults who have been out of the labour market for a lengthy period. Job descriptions are more fluid and firms, focusing on 'core competencies', have hived off entry-level jobs to other organisations that once were routes to secure positions. Increasingly the networks to which low-skilled workers and prospective employers belong fail to intersect. As a result it is increasingly clear that excluded individuals, whether through low income or discrimination, no matter how highly motivated, cannot on their own reconstruct and negotiate a map of job finding connections. Finding a job is no longer an individual transaction where a person simply acquires skills and then joins a job queue, where they are individually assessed without other intermediaries being taken into consideration.

Creating new networks of either kind or bolstering existing ones offers a fertile field for practice. Network mapping, capitalising on existing strengths within networks for getting by, creating new networks around existing points of service such as family centres and schools, or by using mentors and volunteers, are all approaches which social workers should be developing to achieve practical ends in their work – whether to provide more informal social care, support people in finding work or help young parents become more effective in managing their children's behaviour. Networks are particularly important when working with individuals that employment gatekeepers view stereotypically as ill-equipped for the jobs market, such as young males without qualifications – black and white – or the long-term unemployed.

An essential element of social work is promoting the development of dependable social networks that fulfil certain functions for people. Networks are not confined to close personal relationships, and they vary in relation to the needs of individual users, but can include individuals, families and neighbourhoods, as well as comprise specific groups of people, for example around types of work or shared interests or predicaments. Moreover, since people interact with institutions, organisations and services, networks potentially include these relationships as well. For a young person coming from a disadvantaged neighbourhood facing postcode discrimination, the network that spans a geographical gap – a network for getting ahead – with information on training courses or jobs or a sympathetic employer may well be a priority. On the other hand, for an older person with no family around, a neighbourhood-based network – a network for getting by – may well be the priority.

The quality, purpose and functioning of networks can vary dramatically: in terms of the numbers of people involved, the degree of interconnectedness and frequency of contact, the quality and duration of the relationships, and the degree to which they are supportive or undermining (Jack 2000: 328).

For practitioners aiming to develop or strengthen a network it is important to recognise what contribution the different social relations within the network will have. Different elements of networks, such as brokering roles, network reach, boundary spanners and peripheral players, need to be identified along with the specific kind of social sustenance they provide. There are advantages in using a simplified network map in cooperation with users that could prompt further information on their connections and supports as well as day-to-day contacts with agencies and other organisations – or the absence of these. The importance of networks should not lead practitioners to regard the business of putting such a map or grid together in an overly formal way. Remember the aims of network mapping: drawing on strengths, getting the big picture, encouraging family members to tell their story and reflect on their perspectives on their current circumstances. It provides a basis for both practitioner and family to discuss the specific nature of a family's networks and highlights potentially useful resources.

PARTNERSHIP WORKING

Partnerships and multi-agency working dominate all aspects of social care delivery. Difficult as it may seem to believe now, this was not always the case. Public agencies were long accustomed to working within their own 'silo', providing services without reference to other organisations. From the mid-1990s onward there was recognition that many social problems required more holistic or multi-agency approaches. Central government funding became dependent on organisations forming working partnerships – first in community safety, health action, neighbourhood renewal and early years provision. This soon extended to integrated health and social care, palliative care and adolescent mental health, each with their own partnership characteristics and dynamics. Now they are found in every corner of service provision from the smallest neighbourhood service to the large-scale. A huge literature has followed suit, particularly in each, with its own evaluative literature.

Early in the development of partnership rationales the many-sided nature of social exclusion and the interlocking social problems that are at its heart strongly pointed toward coordinated, joint approaches across a range of services such as housing, welfare, education and youth services.

Some of the positive outcomes through partnerships include joint problem solving, distribution of responsibility, and developing a multi-pronged approach to difficult social problems. Professionals find multi-agency activity stimulating, with increased knowledge, but also increased uncertainty about their professional identities and concern about increasing demand on their services. Empirical evidence for impacts on service users, however, is sparse, with some evidence of speedier and more appropriate referrals (Atkinson *et al.* 2007).

Partnership discourse implies some kind of working agreement, tacit at least if not explicit. Partnerships may be founded on unequal distribution of power among the partners who nevertheless come together to achieve a common objective that may or may not be made explicit in a formal arrangement. They come in all shapes and sizes, bringing together user groups with local authority staff, charitable and community sector organisations along with for-profit providers. Users and their advocates, demanding a greater say in decisions, and digital technology are two catalysts for increased partnership working. Years of austerity have shaken the world of service provision – reducing the once influential leadership role of local authorities in partnership formation on the one hand while augmenting the role of charities and private companies on the other, as local authorities and government outsource or divest themselves of services. Open markets for services have transformed social care provision, especially for adults, but also early years provision, bringing capitalist incentive structures into services which had for decades, and however imperfectly, been based on collective ideals.

Partnership formations embrace so many disparate entities that it is difficult to categorise them accurately. Attempts to distinguish between partnership, alliances, networks, collaborations, forums, consultation and multi-party working groups foundered on overlapping definitions and imprecise criteria (Glendinning *et al.* 2002). One set of researchers saw that efforts to categorise them might well be exploited politically – a 'disciplinary mechanism to determine who gets funding, recognition and support' (Larner 2006: 59) – allowing all kinds including partnerships of mere convenience or paper partnerships. On the other hand it is possible to track the *intensity* of partnership arrangements on its constituent organisations. How far is a partnership commitment influencing the work of the organisation? How far is it largely a matter of signing up to a joint language? How far have aims and objectives had to be changed?

Multi-agency working to some extent overlaps with partnership definitions but often retains a more informal arrangement, coming together for specific tasks such as safeguarding. Key questions to ask about any multi-agency working are: Are there organisational structures set up to support multi-agency working? To what extent are agencies and/or professionals working towards a shared vision or common goal? To what degree are services synthesised and coordinated? To what extent is the focus of services on the service user? (Atkinson *et al.* 2007).

The environment in which partnerships are formed is always changing and currently is characterised by loss of a central agent – the local authority. Fragmentation of service environment is characterised now by competing markets, entry of start-ups, both private and social enterprises, various community groups, public agencies in reduced capacity, spin-offs and outsourcing. Local facilitators in the form of parish councils, volunteers and community brokers increasingly have to shoulder complex sophisticated organisation tasks and exercise new forms of leadership and management skills. Partnership formation often embraces new and idealistic organisations in partnership with financially strapped local authorities to provide a critical service, especially in adult social care and youth services. These new entities are then expected to introduce new ways of working, build new relationships, create supportive environments, demonstrate cultural sensitivity – a workload built on hope, volunteers and relatively slender resources that can lead to over-commitment and stress on the part of staff and volunteers (Hamer 2006: 59).

Partnerships *per se* do not guarantee successful outcomes and at times they may be worse than no partnership at all. They may exist only on paper simply to provide a smokescreen for capturing resources. Individual organisations in a partnership may have vastly different levels of influence, allowing dominant agencies to smother the interests of smaller, often community-based organisations. Centrally imposed conditions for competitive bidding carry their own drawbacks. They often stipulate a short time-frame for submitting applications, giving considerable advantage to those larger agencies with a specialised workforce and the capacity to undertake the hours of necessary planning and report writing that grant applications require. Local organisations, community groups, users and local residents usually have no such resources to fall back on, so for them to enter into a partnership on equal terms can be difficult.

LEARNING WITHIN PARTNERSHIPS

* A learning culture within the partnership fosters openness and deliberation, placing large and small partners on equal footing.
* Discussions throughout the partnership mediate conflicting interests and competing philosophies, and how these influence the process of knowledge building.
* Link shared learning to change within constituent organisations.
* Sustain investment to develop ways of facilitating peer-to-peer and organisational learning.

(adapted from Coote *et al.* 2004: xiv)

Partnership effectiveness

In creating effective partnerships there are a number of things for practitioners to think about:

* Make sure that any issues from past activity are aired among would-be partner organisations. From these discussions one can begin the process of identifying future positive behaviours, redefining roles and changing the language from the politics of agency self-interest to the mutual responsibility of partnership. The

biggest gap to be bridged in any partnership involving local people is between the professional and their interests.

- Become familiar with the 'turf' and core interests of would-be partners; few partnerships are agreed without some losses as well as gains for all parties.
- Establish a number of joint problem-solving teams to identify solutions. While holistic or joined-up services are the aim, the path is strewn with practical difficulties both small and large. The advantage of smaller problem-solving teams is that in the more informal atmosphere the 'sacred cows' can be discussed and all parties become involved in the identification of problems and in generating the solutions to overcome them (Anastacio *et al.* 2000).
- Joint problem solving provides the ability to debate the issue in purposeful ways without resort to traditional blocking-type tactics.
- Action learning – an action team of a dozen people can be useful in exploring complex problems. It may choose to acquire expert assistance and policy specialists or conduct study visits and seminars.

Effective partnerships reflect a state of mutual trust and respect that has to be earned. As the behaviours, language and spirit of the new relationship emerge, the competence of each participant is tested and established. To create a partnership without strong foundation is merely a declaration of friendship, or a short-term measure that will struggle to survive the challenges facing it (Sabel 1993). Developing trusting working relations takes time among agencies who may have competing interests. Collaboration is not easy for competitors. The single biggest drawback to the partnerships in government-promoted initiatives is the short time-frame for forming partnerships which must be done before proposals can be submitted.

REFLECT AND DECIDE: POWER WITHIN PARTNERSHIPS

Knowing how power works within a partnership is critical. When trying to understand where power and influence lie within a partnership that you are familiar with, list the agencies and organisations involved and, on a scale of 0 to 5, rate the degree of power that each holds within the partnership (with 5 as the highest). What are the reasons and what is the basis for the degree of power that each organisation holds? Have the power relationships changed over time and if so why? What are the key characteristics of the power relationships of that particular partnership?

> ### CASE STUDY: MENTAL HEALTH CARE IN LAMBETH – A CONTRACT-BASED PARTNERSHIP
>
> With high rates of mental health problems among residents, commissioning a responsive mental health service was a high priority for the local authority and the NHS. The approach taken in 2012 was to form an 'alliance contract' which brought together the council, the Lambeth clinical commissioning group, GPs, service providers in the form of hospital and NHS foundation trusts, and voluntary and community sector organisations involved with the homeless and social care. All providers, under the single contract, submitted to a single performance framework aligned to objectives and shared risks. Incentives in the contract focused on rehabilitation and recovery of service users rather than on existing assets and services. All partners have an equal stake in getting people well.
>
> The aim of the contract was to move away from heavy investment in high-cost, bed-based provision to provision that supported people in their own homes and neighbourhoods. This was achieved by providing early help through personalised care and support – combining cost savings with better outcomes for individuals.
>
> Some of those savings are to be invested in early intervention and preventive services overseen by Lambeth Living Well Collaborative – the providers' group within the alliance that focuses on 'co-producing' services with users. This is a resource centre for information and peer-to-peer discussions and the use of personal budgets – for home visitors, counselling, skills training, telephones.
>
> (adapted from O'Rourke 2015)

PROMOTING PARTICIPATION

Ensuring that users are included in discussing, planning and arranging the services that will affect them is the fourth essential element in any practice aimed at reducing exclusion. Historically both central and local government designed top-down services that relied on a notion of infallible professional expertise tied to bureaucratic procedures that followed certain, often hidden rules. This only reinforced a sense of powerlessness even when the aim was ostensibly in alliance with those they served. For users not to be involved is itself exclusionary.

A long and vital march by advocacy groups in the first instance, and then among various agencies, social work educators and finally government itself, urged direct involvement of users in the decision-making apparatus that allocates resources and designs policy and practice. In some thirty years the ground has shifted to the point that – at least in the discourse of participation – the user is to be involved at all levels of decision making across the entire range of social services but particularly adult social care.

People participate from different motives but all participation involves taking action of some kind that will have consequences (for themselves or society) and being part of something even when the action is individual; all who participate want to do something that is worthwhile in their own terms (Brodie *et al.* 2011). A recent National Council for Voluntary Organisations survey grouped participation into three main categories:

1   *Social participation*: the range of activities that individuals are involved in. These include formal roles in voluntary organisations such as working in a charity shop or acting as a trustee, informal roles with a local association such as a garden club, and engagement in mutual aid – a self-help or peer support group.
2   *Public participation*: individuals engaged with the structures and institutions of democracy – taking part in consultations, contacting political representatives, applying pressure through lobbying or demonstrations.
3   *Individual participation*: the individual's actions and choices reflect the kind of society they want to live in – buying or boycotting particular products, recycling, giving to charity, helpful gestures such as visiting a neighbour (National Council for Voluntary Organisations 2011).

Bogus empowerment

The question of whether participation is empowering – actually enables the relatively powerless to make an impact on decisions, exert influence, engage in meaningful dialogue with those in power and authority – is as relevant as ever. Arnstein's famous ladder (1969) and its many imitators distinguished the authentic from the bogus forms of empowerment (see Figure 3.2). Empowering others, according to Ciulla, means doing one of the following: 'you help [people] recognize the power that they already

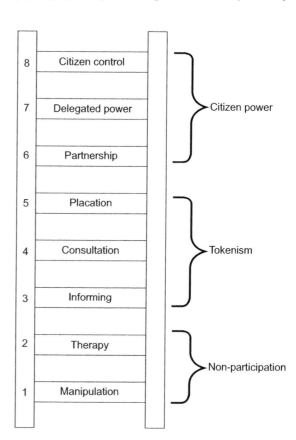

FIGURE 3.2   Arnstein's ladder of participation (Arnstein 1969)

have, you recover power that they once had and lost, or you give them power that they never had before' (Ciulla 2004: 60). She argues that authentic empowerment entails a distinct set of moral understandings and commitments between those leading the process and those being empowered. The moral concepts she has in mind are responsibility, trust, respect and loyalty. They are reciprocal, 'that is, they exist only if they are part of the relationship between followers and leaders'.

> When leaders really empower people they give them the responsibility that comes with that power. Empowerment programs that give employees [or local people] responsibility without control are cruel and stressful. Authentic empowerment gives employees control over outcomes so that they can be responsible for their work.
>
> (Ciulla 2004: 78)

With this near universal endorsement of participation, or at least the discourse of participation, have come fundamental problems. User involvement and participation are poorly defined terms, meaning different things to different people. They are contested, misused, co-opted (Beresford 2012). User involvement has been framed within a market economy, concludes Beresford, and within a service environment whose operation and values reflect the market place. At the same time austerity and front-line service cuts have only further reduced the scope of choice.

Although users are able to choose their services they do so within a consumer model that commodifies need with user involvement based on the resources that individuals have at their disposal – direct payments, personalised budgets and self-directed support – rather than on collective provision based on rights, entitlements and pooled risk (Beresford 2012: 26). This is a central contradiction that appears again and again: the invitation to involvement running up against the realities of market-based provision. Where once it was ultimately the local authority that one could challenge or protest to over, for example, a tokenistic consultation, a fragmented system of social care, with funding and power also fragmented and dispersed, accountability for the involvement process is far more elusive.

CASE STUDY: INVOLVEMENT AND ENGAGEMENT – DEVON COUNTY COUNCIL

The duty to consult users has been widely embraced with councils establishing involvement and equalities teams. Devon County Council has established an Engagement gateway, the point at which users – older people, children and young people, carers and those with disability – have their say on current service delivery and plans for service development. Questionnaires, focus groups on specific topics, expert panels, web surveys, reports back and results analysis are all used to gather opinion. The Involvement team is also responsible for ensuring that commissioning throughout the authority undertakes requisite consultation prior to awarding contracts, and assesses the impact in terms of the Equality Act 2010 (Bird and Simkin 2014).

User involvement is not automatically an inclusive process. Who gets to be involved is a critical question as mainstream user groups are generally favoured over organisations representing marginalised groups such as hate crime victims, asylum seekers, people in residential care, people on low incomes or those who are lesbian, gay, bisexual or transgender. There is a conflict between the consumerist model and self-advocacy movements of service users asserting rights to voice, agency, inclusion in deciding 'who gets what when and where'. Redistribution of power lies at the heart of these battles over participation while divisions are masked by a common language of 'involvement' (Beresford 2012: 28).

CASE STUDY: COUNT ME IN TOO

'Count Me in Too' in Brighton provides an example of the years of hard work harnessing the energies of the LGBT community together with academic researchers and community organisers. It has worked on behalf of LGBT people in partnership with mainstream agencies such as police, drugs and alcohol action teams and the city council. It further developed as a collaboration of the disenfranchised to include deaf and disabled people, travellers, hate crime victims and sex workers, among many (Browne et al. 2012).

Citizens of lower social and economic status are at a disadvantage when it comes to participating in local affairs. They have to struggle against experiences that tell them that government is really not much concerned with their interests and aspirations and that the public sphere is open to citizens 'by invitation only' (Schier 2000). Voluminous studies on participation in the US have shown the disparity in levels of participative activity according to income (Schlossman et al. 2013). The public sphere at all levels and across all sectors is dominated by upper-income-bracket professionals possessing specialised knowledge and who understand the process and the coded language through which public points are made to stick. Organised interest groups, capable of marshalling impressive amounts of money and expertise, shape policy in favour of those interests, while those groups without such resources need to grapple hard even to get a place at the table, and even harder to be heard and have their voice respected.

WORKING AT NEIGHBOURHOOD LEVEL

We have come to know much more about how the social and organisational characteristics of neighbourhoods affect the lives of all who live there. Health inequalities, ethnic segregation, overcrowding and its consequences, degree of physical abuse – all have a correlation with 'place'. Place of residence is strongly configured by level of income and ethnicity which together influence both the physical (or built) environment and the social environment. The first includes transportation, street design, public spaces and access to resources such as healthy foods and leisure opportunities. The second – often referred to as 'social capital' – includes social connections between neighbours, social norms, the level of trust, feeling of safety (or otherwise) and associational life.

Together they are determinate of the health and wellbeing of individuals (Diez Roux and Mair 2010).

The accumulated social capital can be positive by providing resources and strengths that far outstrip anything that professional services could offer. Neighbourhoods with high levels of civic activity such as volunteering, thriving parent–teachers associations, running community halls or neighbourhood watch schemes, are likely to participate in community projects at higher rates with, for example, greater willingness and skills to serve on management boards and committees. On the other hand, neighbourhoods may have destructive effects on residents with threats such as high crime, non-existent job opportunities and poor schools. Few individual families have the resilience to surmount these threats on their own (Wilson 1996; Sampson 1999). Neighbourhoods can also be 'closed' in their affiliations, hostile to diversity, a seed bed for hate groups and physical attacks. Either way the importance of neighbourhoods cannot be ignored. The spread of 'locality teams' and neighbourhood-based teams among service providers is recognition of this fact.

Cutbacks in local authority spending have increased the need for communities to develop their own service projects as council-provided services reduce significantly. Yet public funding that community organisations can draw on and the grants available for volunteer projects of all kinds are substantially reduced. This general trend in policy has placed an enormous load on what has been described as the 'civic core' of communities – those individuals who regularly volunteer in civic life, powering parish councils, school governing boards, volunteer fire services, volunteer youth services, home visiting schemes, community hall management and so forth.

WHAT IS A NEIGHBOURHOOD?

Neighbourhoods may have definable features such as railway tracks, highways or rivers, but more likely form around a specific type of housing, a set of shops, or streets with similar characteristics. Although they may have common features 'neighbourhood' remains a flexible and diverse concept. Some definitions are based on 'walkable distance', for instance – but people with disability could well take a different viewpoint on what they consider to be their neighbourhood. Political entities such as wards or constituency boundaries can be important in defining a neighbourhood but so can attendance at specific churches, mosques, temples and synagogues. Neighbourhoods may or may not have a common feeling of 'community' in which residents perceive certain common interests that arise because of their relative proximity.

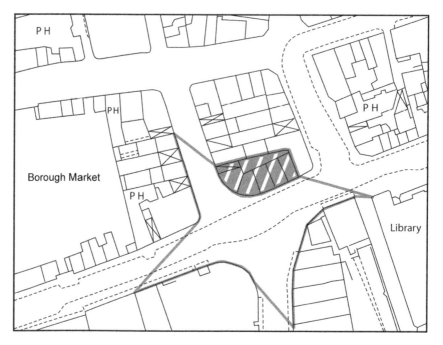

FIGURE 3.3   'Eyes on the street' (author)

'EYES ON THE STREET'

An example of a positive neighbourhood effect is highlighted by the strength of informal mechanisms by which residents achieve some degree of informal social control. These include the monitoring of spontaneous play among children, a willingness to intervene to prevent acts of intimidation by teenage peer groups, and confronting persons who are exploiting or disturbing public space. The capacity of residents to control group-level behaviours is an important dimension to the social environment.

The late urban specialist Jane Jacobs coined the phrase 'eyes on the street' to summarise this capacity of informal social control and how it could easily be disrupted by the poor planning of unthinking bureaucrats (see Figure 3.3). Older neighbourhoods that had physically developed over time presented far greater opportunities both physically and socially for the public to stay involved in the social life of the neighbourhood.

While social work is often, and rightly, described as individual- and family-oriented, particularly in its approach to statutory work, it has to some extent taken a 'neighbourhood turn', particularly in relation to children's wellbeing, with the emphasis on ecologically based assessment, early years foundation and 'preventive' services in general (Holland *et al.* 2011). Adult neighbourhood-based services have also moved forward in relation to mental health, dementia care, and 'ageing in place'. Holland *et al.* (2011: 703) urge social work researchers and practitioners to investigate the interrelationship between neighbourhoods and wellbeing (or lack of it). If phenomena such as adolescent mental health or substance use are spatially clustered, then methods that are 'spatially aware' will expand the evidence base for practitioners, pointing them toward community-level targets for practice, as they come to more fully understand the impact of communities on individual assessments of need and risk.

KEY POINTS

The chapter has explored the five building blocks for a practice that aims to combat social exclusion:

- ❏ The importance of focusing on income and of having a broad working knowledge of the benefits system as a whole.

- ❏ The contribution that networks make both as a professional tool and as a source of social support for users.

- ❏ Partnerships with other service agencies and local organisations through which holistic, 'joined-up action' is delivered on the ground.

- ❏ Benefits and difficulties in building high levels of user and resident participation.

- ❏ The importance of 'neighbourhood' and strengthening local capacity through service approaches to community development.

KEY READING

Danny Burns and others, *Making Community Participation Meaningful* (Policy Press, 2004). A practical handbook on participation.

Peter Beresford and Sarah Carr, *Social Care, Service Users and User Involvement* (Jessica Kingsley Publishers, 2012). Casts a critical but not dismissive eye on how user involvement is evolving.

Child Poverty Action Group, *Handbook on Benefits and Tax Credits* (latest annual edition). An essential reference.

CHAPTER 4

WORKING WITH SOCIALLY EXCLUDED CHILDREN AND FAMILIES

THIS CHAPTER COVERS

- The impact of poverty and social exclusion on the lives of children and their families.

- The ecological approach to tackling exclusion.

- Assessing children in need.

- Early intervention with families with multiple disadvantages.

- Safeguarding and exclusion.

- Children with disability.

This chapter brings together the evidence showing the impact of poverty and social exclusion on families and in particular how austerity has changed the conditions in which exclusion of families can be tackled. Overall it builds on certain fundamentals discussed in the previous chapter: first, that children's exclusion emerges from large-scale patterns of deprivation, and second, ways for practitioners to bring community resources and family resources together in the course of meeting their professional and statutory obligations.

SOCIAL EXCLUSION OF FAMILIES WITH YOUNG CHILDREN

The standard claim from government – that 'worklessness' is the major cause of poverty – is incorrect in relation to children. In 2014 most children in poverty, some 2.2 million, were living in a working family. Of these, 850,000 were in a family where all adults were in paid work, while 1.3 million were in families where one adult was in work. The remaining 1.4 million children in poverty lived in a family in which no one worked (MacInnes *et al.* 2014). The greatest concentration of child poverty – those areas with the highest percentages of children in poverty – was found in the large cities, or areas of large cities: for example, in London, Tower Hamlets 49 per cent, with Hackney and Newham not far behind. In Manchester 39 per cent of children lived in poverty, and in Birmingham the figure was 37 per cent. Liverpool, Glasgow, Hull, Cardiff, Derry and Newcastle were all above 30 per cent. Coastal towns were also affected – Thanet 30 per cent, Scarborough and Gateshead more than 25 per cent.

A significant reduction in the proportion of children living in poverty had been made in the first decade of the twenty-first century, following introduction of family tax credits and other benefit changes. As one authority put it: 'Comparing child poverty in 2006 to its level in 1999, no country in that group [of developed nations] experienced a fall in child poverty comparable to that seen in Britain' (Waldfogel 2010: 136). That reduction has not continued – the Institute of Fiscal Studies and others predict that with changes to welfare benefits the proportion of children in poverty will again start to rise, reversing all the earlier gains (Brewer *et al.* 2011; Bradshaw and Main 2014).

HOMELESS FAMILIES AND THOSE IN TEMPORARY ACCOMMODATION

The number of homeless families housed in bed and breakfast accommodation increased more than 300 per cent between 2010 and 2015.

Nearly 49,000 families in England lived in temporary accommodation in 2015, a rise of 25 per cent in five years; in those families are over 93,000 children.

Nearly half of families in temporary accommodation are led by single mothers.

(Department for Communities and Local Government 2015)

Impact on children

The consequences for children living in poverty are immense. We know that poverty experienced by a child is likely to ripple throughout that person's life. Children brought up in poverty tend to:

* be socially excluded as adults and in particular to remain on low income throughout their lives

- incur health penalties at every stage of their life cycle, with tendencies to low birth weight and respiratory diseases in their early years, and with obesity, heart disease and diabetes in later life
- be more likely to have mental health problems
- experience educational disadvantage as the cumulative effect of poverty on schooling widens the gap between the excluded child and the rest year on year (Hirsch 2008: 4–5).

Families which sustain economic distress often cope also with social consequences – isolation, overcrowded households, children's difficult behaviour, drug abuse and psychiatric disorders (Weatherburn and Lind 2001). Maternal depression is proportionately greater in impoverished households – nearly twice as great in the lowest compared to the highest income group (Spencer and Baldwin 2005: 11). Chate and Hazel (2002) found that the daily battle with tight budgets, debt and overcrowded accommodation brought high levels of anxiety. Only a small proportion of the families they surveyed could buy the necessities for their children that most families took for granted. The most disadvantaged families had higher incidence of chronic conditions such as asthma and illnesses such as acute infections and pneumonia, bronchitis and

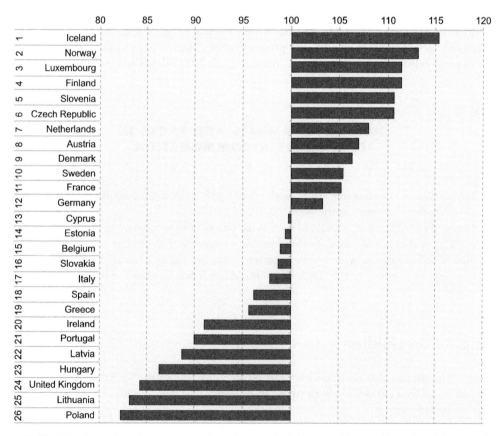

FIGURE 4.1 An index of the material wellbeing of children in Europe (from Bradshaw and Richardson 2009; reproduced with permission from Springer Publications)

tuberculosis, as well as behavioural difficulties in their children – conduct disorders, anti-social behaviours, hyperkinetic disorders (ADHD) and other emotional disorders.

While lone-parent families are viewed as vulnerable, and lone parenting a 'risk factor', all the evidence suggests that it is not family structure *per se* that is critical but the level of income poverty that the family experiences. Jonathon Bradshaw's exhaustive study of child wellbeing across the developed world clearly shows that the number of lone parents in Sweden for example is equally as large as in the UK but that levels of child wellbeing are far higher, largely because of the quality of support services available and the higher levels of income lone-parent families receive (Bradshaw and Richardson 2009). In the UK, on the other hand, a number of factors come together to make lone parenthood difficult (Graham 2013): low pay, job insecurity leading to episodes of 'between jobs', and debt arising from non-payment (or overpayment) of tax credits, and lack of child support (64 per cent of lone parents receive no maintenance). As women form the greater proportion of low-paid and part-time workers, they and less well-off couples who earn below the conditionality threshold will be the first to face the new welfare regime under UC.

REDEFINITION OF CHILD POVERTY UNDER THE CONSERVATIVE GOVERNMENT

The Child Poverty Act 2010, passed by the outgoing Labour administration of that year, set out different ways to measure child poverty combining the measures of relative poverty with measures of material deprivation. On coming to power in 2015 the Conservative government ignored the definition of poverty in the 2010 Act and proposed to measure poverty in terms of family breakdown, educational failure, addiction, debt and especially worklessness. In this scheme, low income became a 'symptom' of poverty and not the cause. The best way to tackle poverty, in its view, was by expanding the job market and not by income support (DWP 2015). The government's proposed redefinition confused what the Children's Society called child poverty 'in itself', that is the brute fact of insufficient income, with the 'drivers' of child poverty – unemployment, parental ill health, insufficient parenting skills and family instability (Children Society 2013). From the point of view of another critic, the new definition of child poverty muddled very different things: measures of poverty, groups at risk of poverty, causes of poverty and consequences of poverty (Bradshaw 2015).

ECOLOGICAL APPROACH TO EXCLUSION

The ecological framework for working with disadvantaged families is one approach that, like social exclusion itself, embraces several dimensions of family life, making visible the many interactions between the child's individual characteristics (genetic, personality, physical make-up), the characteristics and capacities of the parents, as well as the wider neighbourhood and environmental circumstances within which the family lives. In a nutshell the ecological framework highlights the connections between family, neighbourhood and society, how each of these is affected by the others and where sources of support and resilience might be developed.

There is the tendency for social workers to focus on parenting capacity and to meet a child's needs from within that perspective, despite the wider problems and pressures that those parents are struggling with (Gill and Jack 2012). They deploy case management to engage the range of services needed by families, but the approach fails to assess or alter 'the informal world which impacts so strongly on families and fails to tackle systematically material, social and cultural impoverishment, despite readily available assessment guides specifying such areas' (Spencer and Baldwin 2005). Family poverty for example is often regarded as a background condition about which little can be done. One study found that family poverty must be severe before child protection workers took note of it, although the practitioners when interviewed recognised subsequently that the young parents they worked with lacked both the basic necessities for infant care and supportive social networks (Mitchell and Campbell 2011).

The ecological approach asks that social workers consider the entire range of influences on a given family and be aware of the interdependence among social environment, economic characteristics of a neighbourhood and family dynamics. Children's developmental outcomes emerge from the interplay between strengths and risks that span the family, peer networks, school, parents' economic and social conditions, and neighbourhood environment. Child development can only be fully understood within these overlapping and interacting social systems (Gill and Jack 2012).

Around any individual there is an interlocking system comprising:

- micro-system of home and family
- meso-system of school, neighbourhood and other local institutions such as churches, clubs and associations
- exo-system through which more distant but powerful institutions and practices bear on the individual's life, such as parents' workplace, local agencies such as youth centres, or public transport.

(Bronfenbrenner 1979)

Finally there is the macro-system – a large field embracing the cultural, political, economic, legal and religious forces of the wider society. It includes social attitudes and values that, although not always articulated in daily life, nevertheless have a large impact on individuals. For example, our images and opinions on gender, older people, HIV, crime and punishment often emerge from the macro-system.

The ecological approach involves: (i) identifying neighbourhood and community factors that impinge on a particular family through data and information on neighbourhood conditions; (ii) developing an ecological practice theory – an everyday model of how to connect child, family and neighbourhood in a way that is transmissible to co-workers and other professionals; (iii) learning how to combine community-level interventions with family interventions; (iv) developing effective multi-agency partnerships which support ecological practice (Gill and Jack 2012: 9).

Ecological theory widely influenced public policy on child development under the Labour governments between 1997 and 2010, evident in the *Framework for Assessment of Children in Need*, Sure Start and the Every Child Matters programme, based on the realisation that child protection could not be separated from actions to improve children's lives as a whole. Nevertheless while ecological theory continues to underpin theorising and research activity it has lost influence within current child welfare practice.

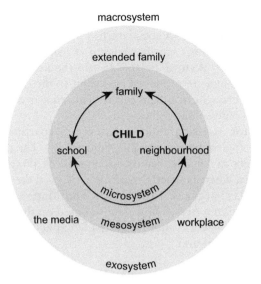

FIGURE 4.2   The child's ecology (adapted from Bronfenbrenner 1979)

Some of the current concerns over the unevenness of assessments of children in need (see below) arise in part because of the inability to understand how aspects of poverty and exclusion impact on parents' capacity for child rearing. Certain areas of the child's social environment receive only cursory investigation, with practitioners focusing instead on the risk and harm from dangerous individuals in and around the family, and allocating resources to essentially reactive responses to conditions that exist within the family (Gill and Jack 2012: 3). Practitioner understanding of 'thresholds' for triggering services is based on the degree of harm or risk of harm and not on a wider view of need (Turney *et al.* 2011; Calder and Hackett 2013).

Assessment of children in need and the ecological framework

The concept of 'children in need' has been fundamental to social work with families since the implementation of the Children Act 1989 and has much in common with children who are socially excluded. Both concepts draw attention to the wider environmental, economic and ecological dimensions in which the child is being raised. Both focus on material poverty, the quality of housing, the child's relationships outside the home and the impact of any disability. Understanding how these two basic concepts relate to each other makes a good starting point in developing approaches to practice that tackle the exclusion of families with young children.

There are differences of course. Social exclusion draws attention to the extent to which a child is participating in society – emphasising that healthy social ties for child and parents are important and that children raised in poverty, without such links, suffer in terms of educational difficulties, poor health or anti-social behaviour. This contrasts with a needs perspective typically expressed in terms of a child's health and development. The social exclusion approach, Axford concludes, maximises inclusion, the other seeks to minimise harm. A social exclusion perspective 'helps shift attention from individualized provision for specific children at risk towards the broader context in which children develop' (Axford 2010: 744). In the needs based perspective economic and social constraints are perceived as distant to the chain of risk causes while parenting behaviour is brought front and centre. This view is widely held and easier to justify politically and professionally (ibid.).

The Framework for assessing children in need (Department of Health 2000a) loosely adopts the ecological framework (see Figure 4.2). 'The third side of the triangle' asks social workers to consider family circumstances along with neighbourhood and community factors, whereas strictly speaking ecological theory would separate the two. Gill and Jack (2012) argue that the Every Child Matters agenda of the Labour government and the Children Act 2004 were also based on the ecological perspective, although, unlike the Framework, that is not made explicit. Among the factors that social workers should look at are:

- the level of local resources and whether the family can access them
- the extent of the child's social relationships outside the family
- the impact of housing, parental employment and income level on the child's wellbeing and the parents' capacity to parent.

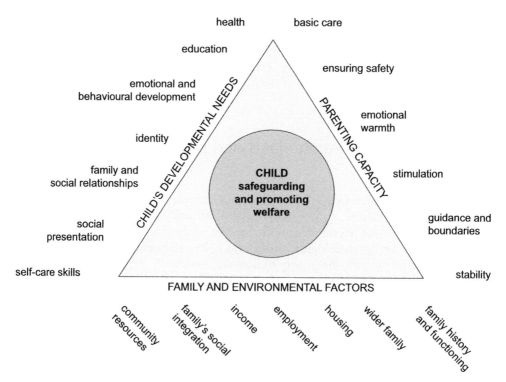

FIGURE 4.3   Triangle of factors for assessing children in need (Department of Health 2000a)

Careful analysis of this interrelationship of the multiple risk and protective factors for each child in need is the key step to exploring the type and level of support to be provided. The different domains of the 'assessment triangle' are not separate areas for investigation and static description but require exploration of their interconnections and interactions in order to provide a dynamic assessment that can respond to change of behaviour and circumstance (Turney *et al.* 2012: 197).

The Department of Health guidance on use of the Framework suggests it be used for collecting information on the child's environment. In the name of 'environmental factors' the Framework becomes simply another checklist. Without an ecological understanding of that environment, however, there is little to suggest that a practitioner should engage with the family in tackling the deprivations found there.

In relation to housing, for example, guidance is essentially asking whether or not the family accommodation is suitable. In fact poor quality housing and overcrowded accommodation is one of the risk factors most highly associated with poor parenting outcomes (Gridley *et al.* 2013: 60). Whether the social worker then engages in helping the family find alternative housing, or sees how the family's housing predicament relates to the quality of housing in the neighbourhood generally, or whether lack of income has meant the family has had to live in substandard housing, is then up to the social worker. There is no direction that she or he should intervene in these matters.

The same holds for employment. The Framework asks whether the family income is sufficient for the child's needs but does not prompt practitioners to examine – let alone assist in – the struggles that parents might have in finding work or balancing work and caring for their children. The first bullet point does call for a sketch of local resources – health care, day care, leisure activities – wrapping up the picture of community-level resources in one catch-all paragraph – with little sense that the practitioner should engage in any community-level work to strengthen any of these supports.

There is a disjunction, then, between assessment that points up parental incapacities and parental failure to meet the needs of the child, where action and case planning are expected to follow, and the 'third side' issues where information is noted but not acted upon. Yet understood in its entirety the ecological model conceptualises a child's needs as multiply determined by forces at work in the individual, in the family or household, and within the specific community and culture, suggesting that these determinants modify each other. 'Thus parental risk factors can be modified by the environment and community' (Gilbert *et al.* 2009: 11, quoted in Brandon *et al.* 2009: 9).

REFLECT AND DECIDE: THE MISSING SIDE OF THE TRIANGLE

Jack and Gill (2003) ask social workers to consider the following assets among others in a child's wider environment when assessing children in need:

- the employment and income of the parents
- the availability of transport
- the extent of reciprocal helping relationships in the community and neighbourhood
- the degree to which parents feel supported in bringing up children

- expensive credit facilities
- the availability and cost of child care
- whether parents feel safe in their neighbourhood.

In assessments of need and in your tacit judgements about a family, which of these factors do you take into account and which do you ignore? What connections do you make, if any, between environmental and neighbourhood factors that an assessment would highlight and the behaviour of children and parents of the family being assessed?

No assessment framework can automatically provide the 'right' answers regarding the needs of children. Ultimately it is down to the practitioner to make a judgement, and professional judgement involves interpretive use of the knowledge that social workers have acquired together with practice wisdom, the sense of purpose particular to them and the appropriateness and feasibility of any action. Assessment is, in Howarth's words, a 'moral activity', a moral decision that practitioners cannot escape making (Howarth 2007: 1287).

SAFEGUARDING AND EXCLUSION

Safeguarding children* dominates professional concerns. Early years practitioners, teachers, youth workers and family support workers are all required to have awareness training on child protection while social workers with children and families must have intensive training. There is bound to be, then, persistent tension between a perspective that recognises, and tries to do something about, the poverty and deprivation in which child maltreatment occurs on the one hand, and the individualised, forensic work necessary to establish whether the threshold of significant harm has been reached in relation to a particular child in a particular family.

Evidence linking deprivation to child neglect and maltreatment

Many studies have established the link between poor material conditions, stressful social conditions and neglect and abuse, and find that families in poverty are over-represented in the child welfare system.

- Spencer and Baldwin (2005) identified the correlation between low income and child maltreatment in their discussion of ecological factors in child abuse.
- Brooks-Gunn *et al.* (2013) looked at high-frequency smacking within families – what they call 'gateway' behaviour to child maltreatment. They found during

---

*As defined in the Children Acts of 1989 and 2004 a 'child' is anyone who is not yet 18 years of age. *Working Together* (2013) makes it clear that the fact that a child has reached their sixteenth birthday does not change their status or entitlement to services or right to protection under relevant legislation.

the period of the Great Recession (2008–9) that smacking rates rose significantly in the US.

- Gilbert and others' (2009) evidence-based review noted close links between socio-economic inequalities and deaths from child abuse worldwide. It also found that poverty, parental mental health problems, low educational achievement, alcohol and drug misuse and exposure to maltreatment as a child, are all associated with parents maltreating their children.
- Golden *et al.* (2003: 106) concluded from their study that parents' 'time, energy and thoughts are concentrated elsewhere in an effort to cope: in this respect the neglected child is part of the family and "shares" its distress and deprivation'.
- Stokes and Schmidt (2011) found that it was the correlates of poverty, such as poor housing conditions, fewer community resources and parenting stress, rather than poverty *per se*, that contributed to increased child protection involvement in her Canadian study.
- UK researchers found that a child's individual resilience in the face of abuse was strengthened when neighbourhood stressors such as crime, poor social cohesion and informal social control were low but not when neighbourhood stress was high (Gilbert *et al.* 2009; Berger *et al.* 2009).

DEPRIVATION IN SERIOUS CASE REVIEWS

The interface between societal issues like deprivation and maltreatment is rarely reflected in recommendations or action plans. These big issues, such as poor environment and bad housing, tend to be thought of as beyond the scope of the review. LSCBs [Local Safeguarding Children's Boards] may consider that these are issues over which they have little influence *even though the potential for a single serious case review to prompt wide-ranging change should by now be understood.*
(Brandon *et al.* 2012: 135; my italics)

There are thorny issues that need further exploration arising from the cold fact that deprivation and low income are linked to higher levels of child maltreatment. Are low-income parents more inclined to be harsh and physically punitive? Is there a causal relationship between low-income status and maltreatment? All together there is little knowledge regarding the possible mechanisms and links; moreover there seems little curiosity in investigating this link. Waldfogel (2000) put forward four possible theories about why this relationship should be: (i) the stress associated with low income leads some parents to engage in harsh treatment of their children; (ii) low-income families are no more likely to engage in maltreatment but are more likely to be reported; (iii) low-income families are reported for neglect more frequently because they cannot afford to provide adequately for their children; (iv) poverty and neglect are associated with abuse but some other underlying factor is chiefly responsible.

Whatever the actual links are, the evidence is clear: an increase in income is associated with relatively large reductions in the probability of risk of child neglect, so clear that it has led the authors of an important study in the US to say that 'there is a causal link between income and CPS [child protective services] involvement, which most likely reflects a causal link between income and physical neglect . . .' (Berger *et al.* 2013).

REFLECT AND DECIDE: IN LIGHT OF THE STATEMENT BELOW, WHY IS THERE NOT MORE EMPHASIS ON DIRECT FINANCIAL SUPPORT FOR PARENTS AT RISK OF NEGLECTING THEIR CHILDREN?

Given that child neglect and CPS [child protection services] involvement impose tremendous economic costs to both victims and society as a whole, this research suggests that economic support policies may be an efficient prevention strategy for physical neglect, and also that child welfare interventions may be well served by addressing families' economic issues.

(Berger *et al.* 2013)

Safeguarding through community initiatives

Whatever the factors behind the association between disadvantage and child abuse it points to a practice that is capable of responding to, and dealing with, deprivation at family and neighbourhood level. Adding to the need for neighbourhood-level response is the greater clarity we now have regarding community-level threats to children, such as the sexual exploitation of children, domestic violence largely on women and girls, forced labour of migrant children, and grooming children for abuse, both online and within some neighbourhoods. These are the kinds of risks that can be missed if socio-economic conditions, the wider neighbourhood and/or cultural context are not taken into account. The scale of abuse in both Rotherham and Oxford offers a prime example that points up the limits to an individual family approach to safeguarding and the costs of not being aware of community networks whether face to face or online. (The issue of child sexual exploitation is discussed further in Chapter 5.)

Community development and safeguarding

Safeguarding is, as Lord Laming said, 'everybody's business', suggesting that child protection was regarded too narrowly as the sole responsibility of statutory services (Department of Health 2003). While encouraging statements were made by the then Labour government declaring that families, communities, voluntary organisations, the media as well as public services all have a part to play, practice based on this principle has been slow to emerge. The paradox of 'community parenting' – defined by Evans and Holland (2012) as parenting carried out collectively or between families within a community – is that it is extensive but hidden. Repeated evidence confirms that parents, particularly in disadvantaged communities, prefer to draw on informal networks* as a source of material and emotional support in whom they have trust because they know the child.

Practitioners have been slow to turn to these networks as a resource for safeguarding children. Mainstream safeguarding strategies continue to follow models based on judgements regarding risk in individual families, while understanding neighbourhood factors that present a danger to children is unfamiliar to many, as is assembling of the needed information. Neighbourhood-oriented practice remains on the margins of mainstream provision, appearing in the form of one-off projects carried out by voluntary organisations or a single team. Yet the connections between the individual family and the social, economic and neighbourhood context should be a central component of any safeguarding strategy. Parenting after all is carried out within a specific social, material and cultural context and is not reliant only on individual skills (Evans and Holland 2012). Pooling the different sources of risk in a given locality and addressing it collectively is the large but necessary step that enables practitioners to bring together initiatives on domestic violence, work with fathers, child sexual exploitation, drug and alcohol addiction, parent management and parental mental ill health, as part of a community-oriented safeguarding strategy.

Successful community approaches to safeguarding can do the following:

- reduce pressures on local parents and children by enhancing the range of activities – play schemes, youth centres, adult education classes, formation of women's groups
- increase sources of informal social support
- reduce levels of mistrust and alienation from service providers
- neighbourhood mapping by children, young people and parents in which risky places are identified
- promote community responsibility for the protection of children – ensure that communities are well informed about the risks to children, and the strategies to protect them
- set up a protective behaviours programme for schools – getting children to identify situations in which they feel unsafe and the actions they could take to stay safe.

(Jack and Gill 2010)

Engaging parents in educational programmes or co-research on neighbourhood conditions can also contribute to reducing the secrecy that surrounds child sexual abuse, and validate it as a public matter that needs discussion, as well as increasing parents' capacity to close off channels for would-be abusers.

Family group decision making

Family group decision making (FGD) extends the concept of the family group conference. FGD relies on committed adult family members, backed by written declarations of intent, to become the primary planning group for the child at risk; it asks them to put into practice their commitment to care for the child by developing family plans to meet the child's needs in the context of the adversity and disadvantage that the family face. Often this will involve other family members – aunts and uncles, older siblings or grandparents – bearing significant responsibility for outcomes, including safeguarding

*Some 30 per cent of children aged 0 to 2 are regularly cared for by grandparents in Britain.

the child. The success or otherwise in particular families depends on the strength of the family network established to carry out decisions taken and its capacity to generate helpful partnerships with professionals that can push forward necessary familial and environmental change for children (Morris 2012).

As Morris has noted, there is increasing interest in utilising family practices – viewing them positively rather than suspiciously – with less emphasis on who or what constitutes 'a family' and more on exploration of how a particular family lives. But there has been little application of this conceptual development when formal state intervention is likely (ibid.). Morris found that kinship placements were 'under-recognised' and only pursued in a formal way without sufficient attention, despite the encouragement from the Children Act 1989. This meant that professional needs to explore family placements were being addressed without a commensurate understanding of family capacity being developed. Given the chance to engage in the planning process, Morris found that families responded differently – they thought more flexibly and showed greater commitment to the child because the balance of power is more equal between social workers and families in negotiating outcomes.

CASE STUDY: C AND HER GRANDMOTHER

I want to care for C full time, give her love and support that she needs . . . she is my flesh and blood and I will do everything to help her. I will take her to nursery or play groups I will go with her to see places . . . I will teach her all the things she needs to know. We all as a family want what is best for C, we want her to learn how to read, write and interact with other kids. I want her to be herself as C.

(child's grandmother in Morris 2006: 24)

Circles of accountability

Circles of accountability extend planning around the child at risk to the community at large. Programmes that aim to engage parents in the task of protecting children from sexual abuse can encounter both reluctance and resistance from families. Which groups within the community will take on this responsibility? Is it possible to engage men in developing protective strategies or is such activity always assigned to women? Finally, how do communities respond to the reality of abuse and abusers once identified?

Such an approach acknowledges the expertise that local people can bring to the task of safeguarding children and establishes channels of communication that can be used to develop preventive and protective interventions. The circles of accountability approach, first implemented in Ontario, Canada, engages community volunteers in the task of reintegrating and monitoring child sex offenders within the community. The approach validates and harnesses the concerns about children's safety shared by many parents and offers a means for communicating about and actively contributing to children's protection (Wilson *et al.* 2011).

Circles are based on the principle that the community is safer when people who have committed serious sexual offences against children are included, rather than isolated, within the communities in which they are resident. Volunteers participating in these schemes in the UK are screened and provided with training.

EARLY INTERVENTION AND TARGETED SUPPOPRT

The case for 'early intervention' – meaning developmental services for children between ages 0 and 3 – is now widely accepted, in part because we recognise that the developing child is learning from birth and in part because it appears to fulfil a number of different policy objectives held across the political spectrum. These include improving developmental and educational outcomes for children, tackling inequality by closing the gap between children from affluent and disadvantaged families, and allowing mothers to get back to work (with reductions then in welfare expenditure).

The Allen (2011) and Field (2010) reports, commissioned by the Coalition government, which largely accepted their recommendations, combined both neurological data and economic benefits to make the case for early intervention. Their findings were in line with research going back two decades including that which preceded the setting up of Sure Start local programmes. A key finding of the Allen report stated that babies are born with 25 per cent of their brains developed; they then go through a period of rapid cognitive development so that by age 3, 80 per cent of the brain is developed. The report made the case for parent support services to improve a child's mental and physical health, educational attainment and ultimately employment opportunities, that will forestall later criminal behaviour, drug and alcohol abuse and teenage pregnancy. Its chief recommendation was to set up a new Early Intervention Foundation – which was duly established.

Critics have noted that the case for early intervention draws heavily on neuroscience, introducing a biological imperative that seems to allow for no disagreement since this is what the 'science' is telling us. They argue that co-option of neuroscience by policy makers has the effect, first, of positing irreversible cognitive difficulties for the under-stimulated child as she or he grows older, and second, pushes practice in the direction of targeted interventions based on family deficits – such as parents not talking to children enough in their first years – rather than toward supports developed in collaboration with the family or improving parenting across disadvantaged neighbourhoods as a whole, as Sure Start aimed to do (Wastell and White 2012). Development in years 0–3, particularly regarding the child's cognitive capacities, has created a sense of urgency in practitioners' views of parenting, making early intervention focus on parental shortcomings while downplaying their strengths and forms of family support collaboratively arrived at.

Others have observed that early intervention has melded with safeguarding issues, creating what Featherstone and colleagues (2014) call 'a marriage made in hell'. The absence of critical scrutiny has allowed the concept of early intervention to drift away from neighbourhood-level disadvantage to search out low-income parents' weaknesses, while the 'parent' focus is frequently simply mother-focused. Indeed social work has consistently shown a disproportionate attention to mothers when assessing parental capacity as opposed to fathers, with much more information about mothers on file than fathers. This is in part because of well documented struggles in engaging with men as fathers and in part because of the unstated belief that women, and not men, are 'hard wired' for caring for children. Of course this highly uneven practice rests on a deep subsoil: the patriarchic attitudes that still assign caring roles in general and parenting roles in particular to women.

The evidence on child outcomes from actual early intervention programmes is mixed: children in high-quality early years settings do show outcomes that last well into their teenage years. However the evidence from early years provision as a whole shows that outcomes fade out over the course of the primary school years, perhaps because the quality of primary schooling has improved. The increase in maternal employment is also modest (Hillman and Williams 2015). Recent governments have sought to invest in child-care provision to create a mixed economy of providers, but in fact the increase in provision has largely come from private, voluntary and independent providers – chains of private providers and not-for-profit nurseries for example. There is strong evidence that the quality of provision is lower amongst private and voluntary providers than in the public sector, particularly in disadvantaged areas where children would have the most to gain. Offsetting this is that children in some urban areas are still able to find public provision such as children's centres and nurseries attached to primary schools where quality is higher (Hillman and Williams 2015; Lloyd and Penn 2013).

Parenting programmes

The case for teaching parenting skills has become stronger over the last twenty years – a product of new awareness that parents mediate the stresses in the child's wider environment. Parenting programmes now work with a wider band of families, particularly recent immigrants, ethnic minorities and parents with drug or alcohol addiction.

INCREDIBLE YEARS

Incredible Years is a basic parent training programme that has demonstrated long-term efficacy when delivered as a preventive intervention with parents of children who show signs of attention deficit hyperactivity disorder (ADHD) and related conduct problems. Follow-ups after the programme was completed showed that: at eighteen months after baseline, a large majority of the sample had sustained at least a modest clinically significant improvement, over half maintained at least a large improvement, and almost a third retained a very large reduction in ADHD symptoms. The results indicated that the greatest magnitude of recovery was observed in those who were in most need, as indexed by having more severe symptoms at baseline. This finding is encouraging given the poor prognosis associated with the condition (Jones *et al.* 2008).

Specific parenting programmes, such as Triple P, Incredible Years, and PATH, are effective in specific trials, but difficulties emerge once they become part of a wider, early years service. One evaluation found that only a third of parents invited to attend a programme provided within a wrap-around early years service did so, and of these only half stayed until the end of the programme – approximately 16 per cent of those eligible. In other words it is not sufficient simply to launch a programme 'that works' – solid recruitment, referral and retention practices are also essential. Axford and others (2012) found that uptake would improve if:

- there is a vivid portal for entry into the programme with where and how to access it clearly and widely publicised;
- there is a sense of ownership across collaborating child agencies, together with an understanding that referrals to it are those agencies' joint responsibility even if each participating agency believes it is already providing a sufficient support to parents;
- outreach activities take place with potential referring agencies, including one-to-one meetings, endorsement by key community leaders at different events, and most importantly, spreading awareness that the programme is not in competition with other services;
- time and resources are invested to train potential referrers on how to best present the programmes to parents.

They also found that parents are more likely to attend if they know and trust the practitioner before the first session, either through a home visit or telephone call, and commissioning arrangements need to build this time in and equip practitioners with the necessary engagement skills (ibid.).

Davis *et al.* (2012) suggest that parenting programmes be practical and clear about which groups of children will benefit and why and checked against the likely group of participating parents. Nor is it enough to expect that parents will just turn up to an announced programme. 'System readiness' requires: (i) a recruitment process, using community leaders with awareness of the programme embedded already in the community at large; (ii) activities separate from the programme that get families interested and keep them interested; (iii) multiple access points – with 'hard to reach' families frequently it is the programmes themselves that are 'hard to access'; (iv) avoiding middle-class bias at all cost, in which a professional lectures a dozen low-income parents, an experience that is disempowering, bringing hidden shame and reinforcing power disparities among those who attend. Most importantly, Davis *et al.* argue that practitioners and commissioners need to become familiar with the psychological, sociological and ecological stress factors that families face and tailor a socially inclusive practice on that basis.

Programmes have to fit in with pressures and time obligations of parents. Time is needed to get all of this right: in Birmingham it took organisers an entire extra year than scheduled to get sufficient families together. Experiential learning, using trainers from the specific cultural community, assisted retention. Peer-to-peer training was found not to increase treatment effectiveness but it did increase engagement and retention in the scheme, with parents reporting higher levels of learning.

CASE STUDY: PARTICIPLE

Featherstone and colleagues give an account of a successful co-produced parenting programme called Participle.

> Workers live alongside the family, persisting through the ups and downs. Interestingly, technology was used by all involved to document and support the process, to record stories of hope, disappointment and resilience. This is a project rooted in today in the use of technology. Professionals are not there to intervene in order to solve problems but to listen, challenge and support a process of discovery and transformation.
>
> (Featherstone *et al.* 2014: 1746)

'Troubled families'

The 'problem family' has made regular appearances in social policy debates for over a century and a half: the family that is so dysfunctional that it wreaks havoc not only on its members but on the surrounding neighbourhood and indeed the country. In the early 2000s the Labour government estimated that around 140,000 families, or 2 per cent of families, were experiencing five or more risk factors from a cluster of disadvantages – the threshold at which child development outcomes are threatened and their behaviour suffers. Those risk factors are:

* no parent in the family in work
* family lives in poor or overcrowded housing
* no parent with a qualification
* mother with mental health problems
* at least one parent with a long-standing limiting illness or disability
* low income, i.e. 60 per cent of national median income, and cannot afford a number of food and clothing items.

(Social Exclusion Task Force 2008)

The aim of the policy response – family improvement programmes – was to provide the kind of support that would re-integrate such families into society at large, mindful of its obligations and responsibilities. The Coalition and Conservative governments have put a new twist on that policy, shifting the discourse from families with troubles to families that cause trouble and deliberately conflating families experiencing multiple disadvantages with families that cause trouble in the community.

In looking for causes of the riots in several urban centres in 2011, the Coalition government calculated that a quantifiable number of 'troubled families' – 120,000 – were prone to anti-social behaviour, largely the consequence of poor parenting.* Such families, the reasoning went, need intensive help to correct their failings; a Troubled Families Unit was duly established in England to coordinate that work with the aim of turning around their lives by 2015. In the discourse of the troubled family there is no mention of ill health, poverty or poor housing. Rather they are a malign force that is responsible for 'a large proportion of problems in society – drug addiction, alcohol abuse, a culture of disruption and irresponsibility that cascades through generations' (Cameron 2011).

The programme is essentially under the control of two government departments – the DWP and the Department for Communities and Local Government (DCLG) – each with its own emphasis: the DWP moving adults into work and the DCLG overseeing family support. Under the programme a key worker takes an assertive, intensive approach to the family, offering practical support as much as two to three times a day at the start (DCLG 2015). The worker's assertive style combines persistence, and the ability to challenge values and behaviour, with an understanding of how the family works as a system. The family knows who their worker is and their relationship is central to progress being made on matters such as off-to-school routines and house cleaning (Morris 2012: 19). While there is a coercive element, with the threat of disciplinary

---

*The final report on the riots noted that there was little if any overlap between such families and active rioters; it used the phrase 'forgotten families' to denote those that were excluded from the mainstream (Riots Communities and Victims Panel 2012).

consequences should families fail to participate, they help those families achieve bet-ter outcomes in health, education and stability, transforming 'anti-social subjects into active, self-governing responsible citizens' (Nixon 2007: 551).

The discourse around intensive family intervention has not gone unchallenged. The problem family becomes a site of scrutiny and governance. In common with most early intervention initiatives with 'family' in the title, in practice they primarily engage young mothers, who are held responsible for the improvements or not that these directive pro-grammes insist upon. Levitas (2012) has noted that the criteria for identifying troubled families were formed in the abstract, on area-level data and not from a compilation of actual families, while the disadvantages that supposedly were concentrated in such families were in fact widely shared by a cohort many times larger than 120,000.

Family learning

There are other less intrusive forms of family improvement. The aim of family learning is to encourage parents and carers – many of whom have previously underachieved and are disengaged from education – to support their children's education and promote engagement with their child's school. It does this by creating occasions for parents/carers and children to take part in learning together. Through specific courses, parents are able to acquire skills – literacy, numeracy, and computer use. Family learning pro-grammes offer routes to qualifications and accreditation, in addition enabling parents to develop the confidence and motivation to progress further (McDowell 2015).

The cross-generational element is important, with better outcomes for both parents and children than if they had separate learning experiences. It promotes the family as a learning environment, building on home culture and experience, and strengthens family relationships and readiness to learn. A wide swath of research confirms that the home learning environment, along with pre-school care and education, are irreplace-able assets (Sammons et al. 2010). Parental involvement in their child's education, both in terms of support and understanding, boosts children's educational attainment (Desforges and Abouchaar 2003).

KNOWSLEY FAMILY LEARNING SERVICE

Knowsley Family Learning Service runs courses and activities at schools, children's centres and community venues across the authority for parents/carers and children. Its 'universal' courses, open to all parents/carers, are aimed at families with specific needs (e.g. parents referred to the service for parenting support, parents who need support with English or maths) and targeted at specific groups of families/learners who may be vulnerable or under-represented, such as teenage parents and foster carers. The range and content of courses and support provided by the service is continually revised and developed in response to local needs/priorities. Its courses

* help parents/carers to be better informed about their children's education and healthy development;

- provide parents/carers with additional skills, opportunities and encouragement to contribute positively to their children's education and healthy development;
- enable parents/carers to re-engage in their own education, gain qualifications/ accreditation and achieve personal development;
- support parents to progress on to further opportunities in education, volunteering and employment.

Courses and activities range from informal, one-session activities, to longer courses leading to literacy and numeracy qualifications or Open Awards accreditation. Informal activities include family reading, maths, arts and crafts, active play, healthy eating, gardening and science fairs. Courses include Family Literacy and Numeracy, Share, Family Cookery, Storysacks, 'Speakeasy' and 'Understanding Your Child's Behaviour'. The service also offers accredited training for parent volunteers and arranges volunteer placements in Knowsley schools and children's centres.

The service's activities are consistently successful in engaging parents with no/low qualifications: 39 per cent of 2013/14 learners had no qualifications and 64 per cent of learners did not have equivalent of L2 qualifications in maths and English. It also engages significant numbers of parents who are unemployed – 61 per cent of 2013/14 learners. Developing more effective support for (and tracking of) progression is a major priority for the service and lies at the heart of this project. However, information gathered from recent provision shows the potential that the service has to encourage learner progression. To date, from September 2012 to July 2014, 67 learners have progressed from family learning on to another education course, 15 into volunteering and 6 into employment (McDowell 2015).

CHILDREN WITH DISABILITY

The Family Resources Survey (FRS), using a definition of disability compatible with the Disability Discrimination Act 1995 and the Equality Act 2010, found that roughly 7.3 per cent of the child population was disabled in 2004–5 (Blackburn *et al.* 2010). The most commonly reported impairments relate to memory, concentration, learning and communication. The steep rise in children with autism, asthma and ADHD presents particular challenges to support systems because of the number of children involved. The study also found a clustering of childhood and adult disability within households, with almost half of disabled children (compared with a fifth of non-disabled children) living with a disabled parent. Families with children with a disability face greater risk of stress, isolation and family breakdown than families whose children are not disabled (Muir and Strnadova 2014).

Exclusion through financial hardship

Families with disabled children are more likely to have lower than average incomes since the costs of raising a child with a disability are more than twice those for a non-disabled child, with heavier expenditure on medical items and toiletries, such as nappies, creams and clothes, as well as items to amuse, occupy and stimulate. Parents' earning power is further constrained as a result of diminished employment opportunities through having to provide greater amounts of direct care for children, while support benefits do not meet the extra costs or loss of earning power. Taken together, households with a disabled child are more likely to be in the bottom two-fifths of income distribution, particularly if an adult with a disability also lives there (Department for Work and Pensions 2011).

Emerson *et al.* (2009) found that families supporting children with developmental delay according to standardised testing at age 3 were disadvantaged on *every* indicator of socio-economic circumstances. Three out of four families had experienced either sustained income poverty, living in social housing, or material hardship (compared with one in three families supporting a 3-year-old without developmental delay). Two out of three children were living in income poverty at age 3. Linked to their material circumstances, these families also had poor self-assessed health and mental health problems markedly higher than those caring for children without developmental delay.

By contrast three out of four children aged 3 *not* developmentally delayed lived in families not in poverty. From his evidence Emerson concludes that the health and social inequalities faced by children with intellectual and developmental disabilities are 'likely, at least in part, to be determined by their poorer socio-economic circumstances and greater exposure to material disadvantage, rather than being inherent in their intellectual impairments . . .' (Emerson *et al.* 2009: 68). In the case of the families with disabled children that Dobson *et al.* surveyed, parents were able to spend only half of what they felt was required to ensure a reasonable standard of living for their child; this particularly applied to children up to the age of 5.

Parental experience of exclusion

The strenuous experience of raising children with disabilities is underscored in a number of studies. Many recent studies highlight the social constraints that impose burdens on parenting. The stigma associated with disability increases the sense of burden. Much of the literature has also focused on the day-to-day experiences of parents rather than their experiences over time and how the needs of those parents and the forms of support they receive – such as short breaks – also change (MacDonald and Callery 2008).

The research into parental stress highlights the social origins of many of the difficulties facing parents. For instance, parents caring for children with cerebral palsy experienced more stress and less support the lower their socio-economic status. An increase or decrease in behaviour problems in children was dependent on income, health and job satisfaction and independent of the severity of the cerebral palsy (Sipal *et al.* 2009).

Other studies have moved away from the focus on the stress of having a disabled child – seen to over-emphasise the negative connotations of disability – to explore the strengths and resilience of the child and family. Generally this research reaches positive conclusions: meeting the challenge of raising a disabled child gives parents confidence in their own decisions and knowledge, allowing them to assert control over their situation, and confidence also in assertively seeking the support they require. Resilience as discussed in this literature is founded on individual traits and family behaviours (Muir and Strnadova 2014). Individual characteristics and beliefs of parents and child of course are important – the ability to be flexible, to have hope and emotional strength sufficient to find meaning in life. Hope in particular – it does not seem to matter what the specific goal of the hope is – is shown to allow a family to adapt to stress events and function in a different way when needed. Emotional strength is also important as the family works together through difficult, distressing times (Muir and Strnadova 2014: 925). The research also looks at resilience in terms of skills and practices – problem solving, developing stable routines, celebrating family rituals such as birthdays, financial management and open and truthful communication among family members.

The research on resilience in turn has its own critics who see it as laying responsibility for coping wholly within the family – specifically with the mother's capacity for coping – paying little attention to the political and social ecology of the family with a disabled child. As Goodley (2005: 334) recognised, resilience has a context; it is 'not an individual attribute, but a product of contexts in which it can emerge'. Resilience, then, is neither a purely individual nor a collective responsibility, less a set of purely independent characteristics than dependent on social resources including informal and formal resources. In their survey, Muir and Strnadova (2014) found virtually all families had hopes for happiness, for their families to remain strong, for the needs of family members to be satisfied and for 'normal' activities such as holidays. But there was markedly less hope when it relied on resources beyond their control. Assertiveness, time-consuming application of energy to obtaining a single resource such as a place at a particular school or to plug a service gap, negotiating eligibility categories for housing, benefits, carers' support, or short breaks, were all part of an ecology that brought satisfactions as well as frustrations.

Disabled children's views

Disabled children in several Scottish studies repeatedly identified their parents, particularly mothers, as very important to them and usually their main source of support. A minority reported that their parents were over-protective, and wanted more autonomy, particularly in going out on their own. Common to all studies was the importance of friendship – as for all young people – and the disappointment in not having friends or wanting more friends. In one study nearly a third of the ninety-one children reported not having spent any time with friends, or having had fun with friends – much less involved compared to a large European cohort of children. Pupils attending special schools often lost touch with friends when they moved to a special secondary institution. While some wanted to meet up with others with similar experiences, specialist support to make this happen was absent, and access to leisure and social activities was curtailed despite statutory duties of public bodies to make information, premises and facilities accessible. Above all, the disabled children and young people felt 'the same' as their peers and had similar interests and aspirations, but were made to feel different in negative ways through what has been described as the 'institutionalisation of difference'. Conversely, some mainstream schools' inclusion policies did not allow for the additional support needed to overcome this difference, suggesting denial rather than acknowledgement of difference (Stalker and Moscadini 2012).

SPECIAL EDUCATIONAL NEED UNDER THE CHILDREN AND FAMILIES ACT 2014

The Children and Families Act 2014 replaces SEN and Learning Difficulty Assessments (LDAs) with a single education, health and care (EHC) plan for children and young people with complex needs. The EHC plan will place more emphasis on individual outcomes and will set out the support children and young people will receive while they are in education or training to achieve those outcomes. Those with existing SEN statements will gradually transfer to EHC plans. The local authority has the duty to identify all children and young people with special educational needs or disability. The Act extends the rights of parents and children to choose the school for their child to young people, now including academy schools, further education colleges and independent special schools and colleges. EHC plans may continue to support young people up to the age of 25 if the council considers that they need more time to complete their education or training.

Ecological practice with children with disability

The ecological approach encourages the practitioner to look at areas such as material disadvantage and local discriminatory attitudes within services as well as the specific needs of the child and family.

Two central elements of ecological practice are: (i) working to make community settings and social networks more supportive of children with disability; and (ii) working with individual families and their children so that they can benefit from involvement in their local community (Gill and Jack 2012). This dual approach is already underway in relation to older people (see Chapter 6), where communities are made aware of, and sensitised to, the needs of a user group, for example people with dementia, combined with social clubs, visiting schemes and social care provision for specific individuals.

A similar process applies to children with disability:

- An issue is identified at local level.
- The precise need is researched and pulled together by local authority or other project workers.
- Local people are drawn into supporting and arguing for a provision to meet that need.
- The benefit of the new provision 'ripples back' into the community at large through support groups, informed local networks and fresh information now available to the whole community.

(Gill and Jack 2012)

Gill and Jack use the example of creating a play park aimed specifically at disabled children who had been unable to access existing play provision – but the model serves for mobilising any new provision that simultaneously draws on the participation of community and individual families.

According to Gill and Jack, families with disabled children require:

- information on services and how to access them, particularly practical services such as child care, short breaks and help in the home
- changing local social awareness around discrimination in transport, recreation and leisure facilities
- focus on the strengths or weaknesses of social networks
- income maximisation.

Short breaks provide for time away from home and parents and were enshrined in the National Service Framework for Children and Young People in 2004. In 2010 the Coalition government included substantial funding for short breaks in its new Early Intervention Grant for local authorities and issued guidance to local authorities (see *Short Breaks for Carers of Disabled Children: Departmental Advice for Local Authorities* (Department for Education 2011); see also Short Breaks for Disabled Children briefing papers from the Centre for Disability Research, Lancaster University). Ongoing evaluations report significant progress:

> Rather than offered as respite for parents the aim is to focus on the needs of the child and enlarging their goals around career, education, interests and activities with friends. A recent evaluation of eight short breaks services found that they enabled children to try out new activities with families reporting that this one objective alone helped reduce their child's social isolation. The same evaluation also found short breaks were effective in seeking out and acting on children's views and wishes in ways that helped children develop new life skills, greater self-confidence, improved emotional well-being and have fun.
>
> (McConkey 2011)

Features of effective short breaks include: ensuring small numbers of children at any one time; a homely environment located in pleasant surroundings; the child looks forward to spending time there; a high standard of care is provided; children are shown love and affection and provided with stimulation and activities; parents have someone to talk to including other parents; transport is available and should be considered integral. Finally, the personality characteristics and attitudes of the carers are as important as qualifications (Hatton *et al.* 2011).

KEY POINTS

❑   A large proportion of children live in poverty, with lasting effects for them and society at large; on current estimates, the proportion doing so will only grow larger by 2020.

❑   Parents in poverty face psychological stress and levels of anxiety associated with the daily battle with tight budgets, debt, and overcrowded and/or poor-quality accommodation. Evidence of outright fecklessness on the part of parents – careless budgeting, deliberately choosing a life on benefits, putting self-interest over the care of children – is rare.

❏   The ecological framework enables the practitioner to see the interrelationships between environment, parenting difficulties and children's needs. There is some overlap between the concepts of children in need and children who are socially excluded.

❏   The practice implications of safeguarding as 'everybody's business' are under-explored. Neighbourhood-based safeguarding initiatives not only address the neighbourhood-based threats to children but also have resources to offer beleaguered families with children at risk.

❏   Families with disabled children continue to contend with exclusion. However, some family services are responding by promoting greater integration among disabled and non-disabled children and young people through social and sports activities or befriending schemes, acknowledging that some young people prefer to be supported by someone of their own age rather than a family relative.

KEY READING

Jacqueline Barnes, *Down Our Way: The Relevance of Neighbourhoods for Parenting and Child Development* (Wiley, 2007). Barnes provides an expert and realistic look at the interplay between neighbourhood environments and children's development.

Deborah Ghate and Neal Hazel, *Parenting in Poor Environments: Stress, Support and Coping* (Jessica Kingsley Publishers, 2002). A still highly relevant study on the interplay between poverty, parenting and stress.

Owen Gill and Gordon Jack, *The Child and Family in Context: Developing Ecological Practice in Disadvantaged Communities* (Russell House Publishing, 2012). The authors are without rival in explaining the importance of the ecological approach.

Jane Boylan and Jane Dalrymple, *Understanding Advocacy for Children and Young People* (Open University Press, 2009). The authors, firm advocates for advocacy as a key social work task, discuss advocacy for children's interests.

CHAPTER 5

TACKLING EXCLUSION OF YOUNG PEOPLE

THIS CHAPTER COVERS

- A review of exclusionary pressures on young people.

- The difficulties for young people in the prolonged transition to adulthood.

- Building relationships with young people and the role of mentors.

- Working with those caught up in anti-social behaviour and child sexual exploitation.

- Working with care leavers.

EXCLUSIONARY PRESSURES ON YOUNG PEOPLE

In Chapter 1 we emphasised how key economic changes have made life choices for young people more competitive, more uncertain and more skill-dependent than twenty or thirty years ago. The impact of these changes has only widened the inequality among different groups of young people in two ways. First, the labour market places a premium on social skills, educational attainment and the ability to handle knowledge and information. Gone are the unskilled and semi-skilled manufacturing industries which paid young men reasonable wages sufficient to establish a family – shipbuilding, manufacturing machine tools, mining, car and steel manufacturing and the like. Second, a results-oriented education system has introduced a curriculum that, whether intended or not, diminishes the importance of trade skills. When government raised the school leaving age to 17 in 2008 it did not in itself alter the structural forces that drive a certain proportion of young people out of education and the labour market. For the roughly 11 per cent of young people alienated from school, this intensive, performance-related environment has made satisfactory educational attainment difficult to achieve.

In general young people are at the receiving end of a cascade of social changes and policy changes that remove public resources from their grasp. The effective end of youth services together with the winding up of Connexions and job guidance in schools has meant that open exploration of concrete work possibilities has largely been closed down – to be replaced by enforced participation in work schemes overseen by Jobcentres and boot camps on one hand and bromides around increasing 'aspiration' on the other. The official aim of careers guidance now is to provide inspiration not practical guidance on career choosing, job opportunities and network creation (DfE 2013).

The New Policy Institute annual survey of social exclusion in 2014 noted that the largest increases in poverty of any group were among working-age adults in the 16–19 age group and the 20–24 age group – 34 per cent and 29 per cent respectively – a result of austerity measures introduced by the Coalition government. In the first half of 2014, 18 per cent of economically active adults aged between 16 and 24 were unemployed, with an increase of those unemployed compared to 2008 of 210,000 (MacInnes *et al.* 2014).

NEETS – NOT IN EDUCATION, EMPLOYMENT OR TRAINING

The proportion of young people not in education, employment or training hovers just above 13 per cent, down from nearly 17 per cent in 2011, with the fall largely from among those most employable. For the half million under-25s who are economically inactive and have dropped out of the labour market there has been no rise in employment. For a substantial minority of those aged between 16 and 18, the high-skill economy combined with a de-emphasis on job placements, and practical and trade skills, leaves them poorly equipped to become independent (Winterbotham *et al.* 2014).

Difficulties in the lengthy transition to adulthood

Many researchers have noted the prolonged and complex nature of the transition from youth to adulthood that young people now face. They have to negotiate a wider variety of routes, with outcomes more uncertain, dependent to a large degree on their individual capacity to actively pursue their interests, rather than as part of a larger collectivity, with virtually no publicly provided assistance to advise and guide (Furlong and Cartmel 2007: 9). While such transitions are difficult for all young people, the notion of 'agency' and 'choice' as to the direction of their lives is more restricted for those without resources, limited not only by material circumstances but also by their exclusion from the networks that secure internships, and entry-level work, and other valuable contacts in securing professional or trade level employment. For those using services, for example young people with special educational needs, a physical disability or emotional difficulties, the transition to adulthood can be brutally interrupted when they 'fall off the cliff edge' at age 18 when in the eyes of those services they become adults (Department of Health 2014).

The focus on individual agency and accountability suggests that success or failure rests solely on the individual, while structural forces – the labour market, inequality of family income, gender stereotyping – are overlooked. Where once the social world was shaped through the prism of class, gender and intergenerational and neighbourhood relations, it is now understood as a field of individual choices and negotiations, mapped against both personal resources and individual feelings about risk (Beck and Beck-Gersheim 2002). Applying for a place at university, for example, requires taking on significant debt and is a far riskier gamble for a young person from an impoverished household than for one from an affluent family. In the same way, when leaving home is triggered by unexpected pregnancy, unemployment or family conflict, young people have to negotiate these problems with whatever personal resources they have at hand without any help from the state.

These social changes require new ways of understanding adolescent development. On the one hand, identity formation is more open, fluid, questioning of traditions. Social scientists have summed this up under the term 'individualisation' – the trend in which the disintegration of guiding social institutions, roles and communal bonds of support compels individuals to make critical life choices on their own, the 'do-it-all-on-your-own biography'. The late German sociologist Ulrich Beck noted that, without the familiar signposts or collective sources of help available even in the recent past, the individual young person faces dealing with risks – and the bets they place on their future – on their own.

On the other hand, the poverty of young people from low-income families restricts their choices and opportunities in ways that are hidden by sociological theories of individualisation (Briggs and Hingley-Jones 2013). The continuing influence of class, gender, place and ethnicity in the biographies of adolescents is overlooked, as narratives of individual pathways based on educational attainment, skill acquisition and work are promoted as the way to success.

The issue for social work is how to make sense in practice of these two different accounts of how adolescents form their identity and their feelings about their lives.

Gender difference

Researchers have long noted how gender impacts on performance in school. As emphasis on numeracy and literacy and academic study intensified, so boys' general appreciation of hands-on learning and physical movement contributed to the rise in rates of hyperactivity. Boys, again in general, regard lessons as arid and de-motivating (Riley and Docking 2004). In the US, girls enter school with a lead on boys, and schools then fail to close the gap. Instead, it increases. The behavioural advantage that girls have over boys in kindergarten, based on teachers' assessments of their students, is even larger in fifth grade. By then, the average girl is at the 60th percentile of an index of social and behavioural skills, while the average boy is at only the 40th percentile (DiPrete and Buchmann 2013).

Boys are also more likely than girls to engage in delinquent acts and bullying, play truant, or commit suicide. Five times as many boys as girls are on the autism spectrum. They are more likely to engage in anti-social behaviour and abuse drugs. There is also evidence that boys are less likely to seek help or to talk about their problems with others. Other observers have pointed out how boys' paramount concern to protect their self-worth creates a fear of failure, with its attendant strategies of procrastination, withdrawal of effort and disruptive behaviour (Jackson 2003).

Girls are more prone to eating disorders, engage in more acts of deliberate self-harm and have a greater likelihood of becoming young carers. They may also have greater problems with self-confidence (Madge *et al.* 2000). It is easy to develop stereotypes – in effect, entrenched prejudgements of an individual's behaviour – around such gender differences and make them seem 'natural' and to miss the fact that each set of behaviours can create a basis on which the young person is excluded from work and community, whether through poor educational attainment, anti-social behaviour or early pregnancy. But the differences in behaviour and in the ways that help is sought are sufficient to raise the question of whether different approaches to working with boys and girls are required.

There has been much recent focus on the link between boys' behaviour and later involvement in crime. The pattern links low parental control and low educational achievement in pre-adolescence with a later tendency toward 'anti-social behaviour' and truancy around the ages of 12–14. In this field there are a number of competing points of view. From the proponents of 'underclass' discourse comes the argument that boys raised by lone mothers are lacking a male 'father' figure and so are able to evade parental control. Feminists on the other hand argue that the upsurge in anti-social behaviour is not the mother's fault, and point to received messages on masculinity embedded in peer-group opinions, media imagery and corporate marketing techniques (Harris 1995).

A third view locates the problem in the economy at large – that young unskilled males are increasingly ill-equipped to cope in school and the world of work. This view points to the fact that vulnerable young men, from low-income families and with the prospect of few qualifications on leaving school, have particular difficulties. Opportunities for these relatively unskilled workers tend to be temporary and short-term, based on sub-contracting or agency employment. They have few chances for training in these casual and insecure sectors and become trapped in precarious patterns that make it difficult for them to secure stable employment (Furlong and Cartmel 2004).

From girls to women

Many commentators have noted the 'sexualisation of culture' – that sex has become a social currency, an ever-present factor in the construction of relationships. Young people are prone to confusion and uncertainty over gender roles; 'sexting', availability of pornography, media stereotypical imagery, cyber bullying and threatened violence from internet trolls have all been identified as contributing to this. Some argue that children, particularly girls, are being pushed into stylised roles submissive to boys at an early age, leaving them vulnerable to male coercion and domination as they grow older. Social media facilitates monitoring individual behaviour and movement, creating a culture of constant 'checking in', with boys using it to control girlfriends. Girls themselves have mixed feelings about the public nature of online interaction that plays all too easily into accusations from boyfriends of cheating and jealousy (Girl Guiding 2012).

REFLECT AND DECIDE: HOW FAR ARE YOUNG WOMEN RESPONSIBLE FOR THEIR SEXUAL BEHAVIOUR?

Melrose (2013: 20) argues that views on girls' victimisation draw on a notion of childhood innocence that is undermined by images of adult sexuality in the media. This, Melrose maintains, pays scant attention to what children and young people themselves bring to how sexuality is defined in their lives and prevents them from being seen as active human subjects. She writes: 'To feel that she is desirable, primarily to men, remains a powerful determinant of a young woman's sense of self worth and identity. It is, for many young girls, the means by which they feel they are worth something.'

This is a debatable statement. Does it accurately reflect gender relations of young people?

A recent survey of girls' attitudes found that two-fifths of girls believe it is acceptable for a partner/boyfriend to insist that they be told of a girl's whereabouts all the time. A fifth said it is acceptable for a partner to shout at a girl and call her names, and a fifth also thought it is okay for a girl to be told by a partner what she can and cannot wear (Girl Guiding 2012). The researchers concluded that from a young age too many girls tolerate behaviour rooted in jealousy and lack of trust, but tend to reframe these as genuine care and concern for their welfare.* Girls told the researchers that they preferred talking about relationships with their peers – turning only to adults when matters became too complicated to handle. They were embarrassed to raise relationship issues with their parents, worried about their overreaction. But comparing relationship difficulties with friends could only go so far if there were problems. In the Girl Guide survey some doubted their friends' sense of objectivity and thought they were emotionally ill-equipped to help when in an abusive relationship (ibid.).

The gay, lesbian, bisexual and transgender movement has brought greater awareness of the complexity and fluidity of gender and its relationship to the sex of a person. Julie Fish (2010) makes the point that a person who identifies as transgender may, or may not live full time in a sex different from that which they received at birth. Being transgender may or may not be linked to gender confirming surgery and, indeed, individuals seen as gender questioning may or may not identify themselves as transgender.

CASE STUDY: ROBBIE

Robert desperately wanted to be female from a very young age. When ten, the family changed her name to Robbie, feminising it to a degree. The following year Robbie started secondary school. While the school was supportive, her peer group who had known her in primary school was not. She was spat on, called names and attacked between classes; in the course of that first year she took several overdoses. Time away from school did not help – the bullying and

---

*These forms of controlling behaviour are covered in part by the new statutory definition of coercive domestic abuse.

isolation only grew worse on her return. Robbie began to self-harm. A transfer to another high school in Year 9 did not work as pupils there had found out. Eventually her parents removed Robbie from school altogether. A place was then found for her at a specialist inclusive learning centre for children who can't cope with mainstream schooling (adapted from Fish 2010).

With lesbian, gay, bisexual or transgender young people it is important to examine the inclusion statements of any institution they may be in contact with – especially schools and local authorities. Do such statements state specifically that sexist, homophobic and transphobic behaviour will not be tolerated? Do staff know exactly what is covered under this policy? What should your response be if you are told, 'this is not an issue here'? (adapted from Beaumont Society, *Schools Out Student Toolkit*).

BUILDING RELATIONSHIPS WITH YOUNG PEOPLE

Relationships are central to working with young people – whether in mentoring, social pedagogy, or the 'reparative' relationship that brings balance to a troubled young person's life. Because a personal relationship is so central, inconsistencies, misunderstandings and feelings of rejection can touch a young person's vulnerabilities, particularly with marginalised youth. Sometimes unresponsive in conversation, erratic in time planning, acting on impulse – these are in fact common habits among adolescents (Coleman and Hendry 1999). But it is important for practitioners to remember that, despite the difficulties and feelings of not being able to build rapport, the young person's interaction with parents, teachers, friends, mentors and social workers has time and again been shown to be the crucial catalyst for young people overcoming barriers of disadvantage. Often the number of adult relationships committed to the wellbeing of a young person will be very few in number – perhaps one, perhaps none.

Much of a practitioner's work will be directly or indirectly involved in creating and strengthening such relationships. What young people value above all is their relationship with the counsellor, social worker or youth worker who is attentive and available. This experience of safety, consistency, trust and acceptance may be their first. For some it may be a revelation: 'I'd never been taken seriously before! He didn't seem fazed! I felt like he was bothered!' (Luxmoore 2000: 74). This goes some way towards balancing previously hurtful, and rejecting, unsafe experiences with adults and gives the young person a broader emotional understanding for dealing with the dilemmas they face.

One of the hardest things for a young person to learn is to distinguish between 'what's me' and 'what's not me' (ibid.: 75). The practitioner's skill in 'reflecting back' – listening to what the young person has to say and then repeating it so that he or she can clarify what they actually feel – is an important tool. Luxmoore cautions against giving indiscriminate praise. A social worker or counsellor should be warm but remain non-judgemental so that young people can begin to discover their own sense of good and bad. Luxmoore suggests, when talking to a young person who feels particularly helpless, asking 'who would understand how you're feeling?' or 'who could speak up for you in this situation?' helping them to identify who is an ally and on their side. Young people whose early formative relationships were destructive need 'reparative relationships' – good experiences in supportive cultures where young people can draw on 'an abiding sense of being interesting and understandable despite all that's happened . . .' (Luxmoore 2008: 14).

Mentoring

Mentoring is a consciously developed relationship that mixes an informal educative role with personal support and encouragement, together with the roles of change agent and advocate. Broadly any mentoring project will 'aim to connect two people in a one to one voluntary relationship, with one person being more experienced than the other and with the expectation that their skills and knowledge will be transferred' (Alexander 2000: 2). Yet how such interventions are supposed to work is not really clear, with the assumption that the mentoring relationship will progressively deepen, reaching the stage where the needs of the young person come into the open with strategies developed to tackle specific problems.

The ideal is that mentoring provides a young person with both a role model – that is, a successful example to follow in terms of a career path, personal conduct or studying – and a source of instruction and guidance. The act of mentoring involves several roles – good listener, critical friend, counsellor, network and coach. Perhaps one of its key assets for socially excluded young people is to provide a bridge to areas of life that have been habitually closed off. This may include useful prospective employment contacts, access to social networks and resources outside the neighbourhood, and guidance on how to make those contacts effective. Mentors are potentially a key element in what is called 'bridging social capital', assets stored in social relationships that are outside the young person's immediate neighbourhood, family and friends.

However, evaluations show that mentoring is a delicate process and only rarely achieves these breakthrough objectives. Mostly it is based on 'ordinary' social interaction with little obvious connection to challenging behaviour or the consequences of social exclusion. The basic cycle is everyday kinds of activities – playing pool, shopping, having a lunch out, bowling. Proactive planning is relatively rare. As one study found, when the relationship does go beyond this initial stage it is often late on in the relationship and in response to a crisis – homelessness, family breakdown, substance misuse, a criminal offence (Shiner et al. 2004). Where schemes have greatest impact is in encouraging disaffected young people into education and work, but in relation to other outcomes – improving family relationships, self-esteem and substance use – there is no clear evidence of positive impact (ibid.).

In order to encourage disadvantaged youth into work, Hollywood and others argue, it is necessary to find what interests young people and then to find those links to the local labour market and recruitment policies that can make it happen. What young people from disadvantaged neighbourhoods need is realism about the labour market and what the world of work is like – such as having to work their way up to positions of greater responsibility. The *reparative* relationship – a relationship that overcomes a disadvantaged background – provides support and encouragement, helps create social networks and provides sources of advice. The Barnardo's Works project for long-term unemployed young people between 16 and 24 years of age adopted this kind of mentoring relationship – including supportive employers who offer a nurturing environment aware that young people are not polished from day one (Hollywood et al. 2012).

Many would-be mentors have idealised notions of what they can accomplish – sometimes encouraged by promotional material that omits the everyday challenges and vulnerabilities of young people. They can become easily discouraged if they view a young person's lack of engagement as deliberate rather than stemming from other factors such as previous abuse or disappointment. Good mentors act with integrity and have the following characteristics:

- Perception of self: do they feel comfortable in front of others? Do they have the capacity to speak about their feelings and are they open about themselves and their experiences? Are they aware of their own prejudices and personal limitations? Do they have a sense of worth? Are they trustworthy?
- Warmth and perception of others: do they believe that people are responsible for their own destiny and that individuals can cope with difficulties when supported? Do they think all people are worthy of help? Are they easily threatened by others and can they challenge others when needed?
- Empathy: do they believe that an individual's difficulties can be affected by both personal and environmental factors? Can they imagine themselves in others' shoes and perceive the mentor's role as enabling and not controlling? Do they respect difference and value freedom of choice?

(Alexander 2000)

Mentors may express beliefs or opinions at odds with those of the young person, show a religious conviction and attempt to proselytise. Would-be mentors require training adapted from counselling principles so that they become aware of the power differentials that are never far away – inherent in the age differences and perhaps in class and cultural backgrounds.

ANTI-SOCIAL BEHAVIOUR

Anti-social behaviour (ASB) by young people remains stubbornly prominent in the public mind and government policy. It is both a product of social exclusion and a force that excludes. Behaviour such as shouting and verbal intimidation, fighting, public drunkenness, vandalism and graffiti often intimidates people and causes apprehension if not outright fear among local people. At the same time those who commit it are themselves often excluded though poverty, from school or the job market.

Adult tolerance of adolescent behaviour quickly runs out when confronted by aberrant behaviour, failing to take into account young people's developmental immaturity, lack of cognitive development or other social and emotional shortcomings. Adolescent psychosocial development is characterised by impulsivity; reliance on peer acceptance, lack of experience of autonomy (and the responsibilities that go with it), inability to extricate themselves from compromising situations, and failure to anticipate future consequences all play their part. To reduce the complexity of adolescence to a culture of control as a way of handling behavioural difficulties is to simplify enormously the nature of the problem.

THE CRIME AND POLICING ACT OF 2014

The Crime and Policing Act of 2014, the latest in a long string of statutes aiming to rein in ASB, defines anti-social behaviour as conduct that:

- has caused, or is likely to cause, harassment, alarm or distress to any person;
- is capable of causing nuisance or annoyance to a person in relation to that person's occupation of residential premises;
- is capable of causing housing-related nuisance or annoyance to any person.

Anxiety about young people's behaviour, particularly in groups, is widely expressed and sometimes encouraged by the media. Defining anti-social behaviour rests essentially on subjective judgement – one person's view as opposed to another's – and on the location where the ASB occurs. Graffiti for instance is sometimes encouraged as public art, sometimes regarded as an offence – it is both an aesthetic practice and criminal offence depending on place and point of view. Over the last two decades the term anti-social behaviour has come to signify borderline criminal behaviour – 'criminalising nuisance' to use one phrase (Squires 2008).

When Millie and his colleagues probed more deeply into what people actually thought constituted anti-social behaviour they found there was concern with just three issues: general misbehaviour by children and young people, visible drug and alcohol misuse and 'problem families' and neighbour disputes (Millie *et al.* 2005). What the public was *really* bothered about was anti-social behaviour as a sign of social and moral decline. The public favoured more disciplinary solutions, while local agencies explained it in terms of social exclusion and deprivation and favoured prevention and inclusion strategies. As a kind of compromise in the three case study sites investigated, each had local strategies in place to combat anti-social behaviour that were graduated and proportional and balanced preventive services with enforcement (Millie *et al.* 2005).

The Coalition and subsequent Conservative government emphasised local solutions that geared responses to the needs of victims of ASB, especially high-risk victims, who are accorded swift response from the police (Home Office 2012). In the Crime and Policing Act 2014 it replaced the anti-social behaviour order (ASBO) and the (housing-related) anti-social behaviour injunction with an injunction to prevent nuisance and annoyance (IPNA). The IPNA covers ages 10 and up with a focus on what are perceived to be drivers of ASB: disruptive tenants, binge drinking, drug use, mental ill health, troubled families, irresponsible dog ownership. It also places emphasis on the nuisance and risk to the victims, who are able to use a 'community trigger' (now more frequently called anti-social behaviour review) – in which councils, the police, health teams and social housing landlords are obliged to undertake a case review when requested and the circumstances meet the threshold. These include the victim feeling ignored or a problem persisting because of an inadequate response from agencies. Local authorities have responded by establishing websites and help-lines primed to receive notice of incidents from the public on anything from unwarranted noise or dogs fouling pavements, to threatening behaviour. But the philosophy of the IPNA also recognises that legal orders do not actually address causes and places increasing emphasis on early intervention and whole-family work of the kind associated with the troubled families programme (see Chapter 4).

Causes of and response to anti-social behaviour

Throughout this volume we have noted competing perspectives on major social problems. Anti-social behaviour is no exception. One perspective locates it as a function of community breakdown, pointing to the lack of informal social controls in a neighbourhood. This lack of capacity to uphold norms of behaviour produces a social vacuum that gives prominence to groups of young people – primarily but not exclusively young men – who in turn encounter no countervailing authority on the streets (Power and Tunstall 1997). A second perspective views anti-social behaviour as arising from conduct disorders in children that may emerge from particular family dynamics. In this perspective the lack of parental supervision, parental rejection, erratic and coercive discipline, marital conflict, parental criminality and weak attachment are all significant predictors of anti-social behaviours, including drug use and offending (Patterson 1985; Rutter *et al.* 1998).

A third perspective links anti-social behaviour to disadvantage and the way public perceptions of young people combine with impoverished backgrounds to constrain choices and reshape young people's own estimation of their future and the day-to-day calculations needed to realise that future. The authors of an Ipsos Mori survey found that it could predict how anti-social behaviour would be perceived by residents in a given area by its level of deprivation, population density, recorded level of violent crime and the proportion of residents aged 25 years and under (Ames *et al.* 2007). A later survey in Northern Ireland pointed to near-identical findings (Cadogan and Campbell 2014).

Practice approaches to anti-social behaviour used by social care and health care staff draw on all three perspectives. There is a link between children's conduct disorders and later ASB. Recent NICE-SCIE guidelines call for preventive strategies involving emotional learning and problem-solving programmes for children aged 3–7, especially in classes where a high proportion of children are at risk of developing conduct disorders: in neighbourhoods of high deprivation where levels of child abuse, parental conflict and parental contact with the criminal justice system are high (Pilling *et al.* 2013). The aim is to promote a positive concept of self, good peer relations and problem-solving skills. The guidelines also call for comprehensive assessment of children with conduct disorders and recommend parent training and foster parent training programmes, discussed in the previous chapter, to deal with 'oppositional defiant disorder'.

There is increasing awareness too of the link between ASB and mental health problems. That such problems are often undiagnosed in allegations of ASB – whether in perpetrator or victim – makes dealing with ASB particularly complex, for example constructing injunctions against individuals within a safeguarding framework. The aim is to carefully weigh the needs of the perpetrator with the interests of victims and communities under the 2014 Act (London Councils 2014).

CASE STUDY: EALING'S COMMUNITY CONTACT REPORT

The experience of the London Borough of Ealing's safer communities department suggested that colleagues in mental health services did not always have a 'real time' understanding of what was going on outside their established contact with their patients. The safer communities department felt this lack of understanding and knowledge was a key factor in how ASB cases were handled, and was an issue that could be addressed and positively influenced.

The council designed a 'community contact report' with the objective to pull together the pieces of the community jigsaw, which cross-referenced all contacts with a family – from homelessness assessment records and mental health records to ASB incidents and police intelligence. As a result, the report could tell a complete story about the person charged with ASB, as well as the nature and degree of their illness and crisis (London Councils 2014: 10–11).

Responding to pronounced behaviour where the young person is skirting the youth justice system, NICE-SCIE guidance recommends multi-modal interventions such as multi-systemic therapy based on the social learning model, with interventions provided by specially trained case managers at individual, family, school, criminal justice and community levels. Not unlike family improvement project work the intervention typically consists of three to four meetings a week for three to five months (Pilling *et al.* 2013).

Theoretical tenets underpinning 'get tough' programmes tend to suggest that youth offending is a conscious act of free will, so offenders should be treated as rational agents who know what they are doing in purposefully engaging in ASB and should suffer the consequences as responsible individuals. This logic ignores the findings of adolescent development mentioned at the outset of the chapter – lack of autonomy, reliance on peer acceptance, imperfect judgement regarding future consequences. Principles of restorative justice shift the perspective, through which an obligation to victims is incurred, acceptance of responsibility for the offence is achieved and work to repair the harm is undertaken, with an evidence base suggesting that this is by far the more effective approach to young would-be offenders (Sellers and Arrigo 2009).

CASE STUDY: BART

Bart, 15, has the habit of intimidating other boys at school. He is tall, wiry and strong for his age. He asserts himself by coming up fast to other boys in the corridors or in recreation areas, gesturing with his fists. When teachers are not looking he will land a covert punch, trip a boy or belittle someone. He regularly uses bad language and can get very angry over the slightest provocation. Despite all this he has his likeable, even tender side. He dotes on his younger sister and was very upset when a local young girl went missing because, as he said, it could have been his little sister.

Bart is on the verge of being excluded from school. As a social worker attached to the school, what approaches and strategies would you adopt with him? Would you try to save his place at school? If not, what would be the realistic alternatives for him? What do you think could be the long-term consequences for Bart of your actions?

SEXUAL EXPLOITATION OF CHILDREN AND YOUNG PEOPLE

As the scale of sexual abuse of children (including any young person under 18) has increased, so has our understanding of its nature and dynamics. As it does so, we can see the profound challenge that mass child sexual abuse presents to the individual, forensic approach to child safeguarding.

DEFINITION OF CHILD SEXUAL EXPLOITATION (CSE)

Sexual exploitation of children and young people under 18 involves exploitative situations, contexts and relationships where young people . . . receive 'something' (e.g.
food, accommodation, drugs, alcohol, cigarettes, affection, gifts, money) as a result
of them performing . . . or others performing on them, sexual activities.

(DCSF 2009: 9)

The definition further notes that in all cases those exploiting children have power over them,
whether through differences in age, physical strength or economic resources. Violence,
coercion and intimidation are common means through which that power is asserted, in
contrast to the child or young person's limited choices because of social, economic or
emotional vulnerability (ibid.: 9).

Sexual exploitation of girls and boys

Sexual exploitation of young women takes several forms: grooming girls in children's
homes and in neighbourhoods, gang-associated sexual violence and sexual coercion
within peer groups. Each in its own way feeds on the wider patterns of masculinity in
society at large and crystallises the pressure and coercion embedded in contemporary
relationships between boys and girls and young men and women.

Broadly, within society's approval/disapproval matrix, young men have the freedom to be sexually active, while young women are judged harshly and are frequently
harmed, reputationally and physically, by early sexual activity. Misogynist attitudes,
contained for example in hate lyrics and attacks on individual women through the
internet, rigid stereotyping of boy-girl behaviour, and fantasies of violence, further
serve to groom the groomers.* Grooming networks and gang-associated sexual violence form the apex of a controlling neo-patriarchy. These are crimes committed by
whole cohorts of men brought together by crude economic interests and gratifications
defined by exploitation, capture and extortion. Although 'rewards' are available –
status, 'protection', money or drugs – to the young women who submit, they are more
likely to recognise the exploitative and violent nature of the sexual contact than the
young men who perpetrate it (Beckett *et al.* 2013). In the report from the Children's
Commissioner, 'It's wrong, but you get used to it', one young woman put it this way:
'*He feels in control of the streets anyway . . . so he'll want things to go his way, so he
won't be thinking "oh this is rape", when it actually is*' (ibid.: 7).

Boys are also sexually exploited. A recent large-scale study by Barnardo's across
England, Scotland and Northern Ireland concluded that boys and young men constitute
a sizeable minority of CSE cases. Characteristics are different – on referral males were
on average slightly younger than females (13.9 years versus 14.6), a greater proportion had a disability – particularly autism, learning difficulty and ADHD – and a larger

---

*There is growing recognition of these trends by women writers. See for example works by Cordelia Fine
(2010), Rebecca Solnit (2014) and Peggy Orenstein (2012).

proportion of males had a youth offending record: 48 per cent of boys versus 28 per cent of girls (Barnardo's 2014b).

There are several pathways into exploitation for boys: through a 'trusted friend', female perpetrators, prostitution, institutional abuse, age-inappropriate contact through pornography sites, and abuse of gay, trans- and bisexual young people. Instances of exploitation emerged through various referral routes, for example going missing (80 per cent of males as opposed to 42 per cent of females), while suspicion of a relationship with an older person, which figured prominently with females, did not do so with males (ibid.).

Safeguarding young people

The failure to protect young people or even to be aware of the scale of the child sexual exploitation, whether through gangs or grooming, arises from ecological ignorance of the hidden networks and specific sites of contact in particular neighbourhoods. Social services have not been proactive in identifying gang-associated sexual violence or exploitation, while police historically discounted child sexual exploitation (*Guardian*, 18 November 2014). Exploited young people themselves are reluctant to come forward. Among those that Becket and others interviewed, only 1 in 12 felt that young people would be likely to report, or talk about, experiences of sexual violence or exploitation, and even in those few instances they would contact a peer rather than a professional. The reasons they gave include: (i) what the authors call the 'normalisation' of sexual violence and resignation over the fact that it happens; (ii) fear of retribution, ostracism or negative judgement; (iii) lack of confidence in services' ability to protect them (Beckett *et al.* 2013: 8).

As we saw in the previous chapter, safeguarding processes essentially rest on an individualised model of child protection aimed at identifying unsafe individuals in the immediate family environment. In this perspective abuse happens by an adult, often within the home. By contrast, in sexual exploitation through gangs or peer-related networks, the danger is in the streets; abuse comes from peers, outside the home in unsafe neighbourhoods. Gang members do not recognise or admit that what is happening to them is abuse but see their activity as unavoidable and freely chosen because it is safer than approaching distrusted authorities. As one expert, John Pitts, has written,

> We can only understand who is at risk, and in what ways, when we have a picture of the social/criminal networks (the social fields) in which they are enmeshed. The people who can do this are the affected young people and their families.
>
> (Pitts 2014)

See Me, Hear Me, a partnership framework initially formulated by the office of the Children's Commissioner, aims to protect children from CSE. It has identified a number of current system failings, among them:

- the failure to recognise sexual exploitation;
- forgetting/ignoring the child;
- failure to engage with children themselves;
- working in isolation among other agencies;
- persistent denial that there is a problem at all.

(Berelowitz *et al.*, 2013)

These are the same deficiencies highlighted by any number of child abuse inquiries over the last thirty years, *with this difference*: the presence of a community dimension that was overlooked by a model of problem identification based on unsafe individuals. A neighbourhood dimension to social work service and an ecological understanding of the forces at work within the neighbourhood would have safeguarded the young people involved. Sexual exploitation of children and young people reached the scale it did in certain areas because social work, and other authorities such as the police, confined their perception of child abuse to abuse essentially perpetrated within individual families. Children, often disabled or from minority ethnic groups, were out of sight when exploited by street gangs and peers, and the wider pattern of exploitation was missed.

LOCAL SAFEGUARDING CHILDREN'S BOARDS' (LSCBS) SHORTCOMINGS IN RELATION TO CHILD SEXUAL EXPLOITATION

Nearly half of LSCBs (49 per cent) told the Jay Inquiry that they did not know how many victims there were in their area in 2012; only 18 per cent could provide data even though 91 per cent believed they had come into contact with victims. Only 36 per cent included children and young people in development of policies and only 47 per cent involved children and young people in planning meetings about their care and protection. They had ready phrases to explain away this poor performance, such as children 'put themselves at risk' or 'not hitting the threshold for statutory interventions' (Jay 2014).

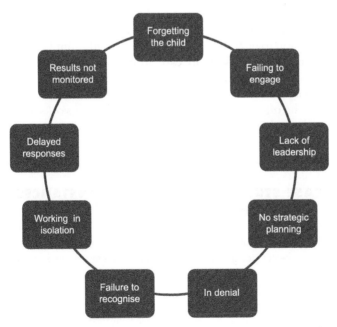

FIGURE 5.1   See Me, Hear Me: system failings (Berelowitz *et al.* 2013; reproduced with permission from the Children's Commissioner)

The challenges for safeguarding at local level, then, are several. Understanding the complex communities in which exploitation takes place is perhaps the most difficult. Developing proactive engagement is necessary – mapping communities, developing specific local knowledge that places problems in context, developing problem profiles. Police in general are effective in mapping criminality, and the health service in mapping local health needs – but mapping exploitation is more difficult since it hides within wider community structures. One of the difficulties in Rotherham was that there was no acceptance that the scale of the problem existed and had no problem profile within the various services. There was awareness within some services, as there certainly was among residents – but 'awareness' and institutional recognition of the problem are two different things. For example, the senior management level engaged in LSCB liaison may rely on a single representative, if any, from different ethnic communities, so detailed knowledge of neighbourhood practices, hidden or otherwise, is difficult to obtain.

Multi-agency partnerships and child sexual exploitation

The multi-dimensional nature of CSE requires a multi-agency approach involving youth offending teams (YOTs), LSCBs, schools and the youth service. Co-located teams improve communication with 'hybrid' professionals – those with experience and knowledge of several agencies, especially their cultures, structures, their terminology and reference points (discourse) and priorities – working across practice boundaries (Drew 2014).

Clearly there are difficult issues for any partnership to work through. How should the issue be approached in public – as an anti-gang agenda or a CSE agenda? Should CSE be defined as aberrant behaviour or is it better to say nothing and cover it over with slogans ('a better place to live')? In general, youth offending teams, despite clear responsibilities to their locality, have been reluctant to press their intervention over fears harboured by social workers and police who argue that they do not know enough about the phenomenon to intervene with confidence (ibid.). But CSE should not be the exclusive responsibility of YOTs in any case. Youth justice is the responsibility of the Home Office and other departments. It is a whole-government responsibility and too often, under national priorities, the work that attracts resources is only those initiatives targeted on would-be offenders and not on the kinds of networks and disadvantaged neighbourhoods through which and in which CSE frequently occurs.

CASE STUDY: INTERVENING IN INSTANCES OF CHILD SEXUAL EXPLOITATION

Police and other agencies are aware that ninety-two young females are significantly involved with Manchester gangs, with 40 per cent of them involved in criminal activity. Front-line practitioners may be wary of working with these adolescents because of the tentative nature of the evidence and the thorny issue of exploring sexual identity and behaviour of young people.

In this instance YOTs should be thinking about diversion. Practitioners are able to offer support for victims to move out of CSE, drawing on public and voluntary services appropriate to the needs of the child or young person, such as sexual health, mental health and counselling. These should take account of both the identified risk factors and the child or young person's family *and wider circumstances*. Previous abuse, running away from home or care, involvement in gangs and child trafficking are all indicators of CSE (DfE 2012a).

CASE STUDY: GROOMING

Two men in their late twenties are grooming six girls – three under 18 and three over 18 – but the practitioner does not know that. The practitioner does know that one of those under 18, a 15-year-old, is not going to school, appears unkempt, and her parents are splitting up. She says to her social worker that she is staying with her boyfriend's family. It is tempting to accept this at face value for fear of misreading the situation. The practitioner needs to find answers to two questions before taking the next step: (i) how old is the boyfriend? (ii) what is the family like that she has moved into? At this stage it is difficult to engage the LSCB because it is not yet an identified child protection issue.

Key indicators of possible CSE: going missing for periods of time or regularly coming home late; regularly missing school or education or not taking part in education; appearing with unexplained gifts or new possessions; associating with other young people involved in exploitation; having older boyfriends or girlfriends; suffering from sexually transmitted infections; mood swings or changes in emotional wellbeing; drug and alcohol misuse; displaying inappropriate sexualised behaviour.

Practitioners should give careful consideration to the issue of consent. It is important to bear in mind that:

- a child under the age of 13 is not legally capable of consenting to sex (it is statutory rape) or any other type of sexual touching;
- sexual activity with a child under 16 is also an offence;
- it is an offence for a person to have a sexual relationship with a 16- or 17-year-old if they hold a position of trust or authority in relation to them;
- where sexual activity with a 16- or 17-year-old does not result in an offence being committed, it may still result in harm, or the likelihood of harm being suffered.

An assessment under Section 17 of the Children Act 1989 must be undertaken in all cases where child sexual exploitation, or the likelihood of it, is suspected. The local authority, health and other partners must follow the process set out in the Framework for assessment of children in need and their families. The assessment is not an end in itself, but the means of informing the planning and delivery of effective services for children. The requirement to make timely, proportionate assessments to understand a child's needs and circumstances is critical to secure good outcomes for the most vulnerable children and young people. The assessment should contain a conclusion as to whether the child is suffering, or is likely to suffer, significant harm (DfE 2012a).

CASE STUDY: AN ASIAN-ONLY PROBLEM?

During a meeting with two health workers, the Rotherham Inquiry team asked about the profile of perpetrators in the local area. It was told that they were exclusively 'Asian males'. The team then asked the workers to talk through one of their live cases. The detail gave a different picture. The workers said the victim had been exploited in school by her peers, who were all white boys. She was subsequently exploited by an older boyfriend who was an Asian man in his twenties. Following this, she was exploited by an older white man who filmed her having sex with his friends. She was then exploited by a group of older Asian men who sold her at parties. Finally, an older white man, who was addicted to drugs, exploited her. He took her to the homes of much older, disabled men, and sold her to pay for his drug habit. These health workers had mentally screened out the white perpetrators. (Example given at a meeting during Phase 2 of the Inquiry)

CARE LEAVERS

The family background of children and young people coming into care is chequered by unemployment, low income from benefits or low-wage jobs, and parental discord. In the large YiPPEE study (Young People in Care – Pathways to Education in Europe), for example, very few of the children or young people in care had been living with both birth parents; virtually all parents were divorced or had never lived together, and most were unemployed, relying on benefits, or in low-wage jobs. Domestic violence, physical and sexual abuse, drug and alcohol addiction, mental health problems and criminal activity were also prevalent in the families (Jackson and Cameron 2014: 22).

NUMBER OF CHILDREN AND YOUNG PEOPLE IN CARE

As of 31 March 2014 there were 68,840 children and young people 'looked after' by local authorities in England and Wales – a number that has increased steadily since 2010 when it stood at 64,470, and higher than at any point since 1985, but with large variations among individual local authorities. Of 27,220 care leavers in the year to March 2014, 38 per cent were not in education, employment or training, while 78 per cent were classed as living in 'suitable accommodation' with 39 per cent living independently, although these figures are undermined by those local authorities who included 'residence unknown' and 'in custody' as 'suitable' (Department for Education 2014b).

In general, parents act as their child's best advocate from birth, knowing that certain choices, decisions and milestones affect their children's life chances. In the main, parents take their children's needs vigorously into account, pushing schools to respond to those needs, advising their child as he or she gets older, watching out for any special needs or health problems. Parents are particularly involved in their child's education: selecting schools, supporting – and if necessary enforcing – their child's attendance, helping to choose subject options, assisting and reminding on homework, getting in touch with teachers if there are difficulties, and advising on work experience.

When a child enters public care the situation changes dramatically. The child, whether accommodated with parental agreement or subject to a care order, rarely has an advocate equal to the commitment that parents in general hold to. Local authorities have a variable record when acting as the parent for children they look after, and for all the focus on the quality of state care and requirements to improve the skills and educational attainment of care leavers in the last dozen years and more, it is remarkable how difficult changing that culture has been. Not until 2007 were the two services relating to looked after children – care system and education system – brought together.

Overcoming the effects of this historic divide is an urgent task. Education is not the sole responsibility of the classroom. Through everyday actions adults are helping young people 'form their values, views about the world and "how to be" in relation to others' (Cameron et al. 2015: 10). The idea of social pedagogy argues that care and education are integral to each other – 'learning placements [in care] and caring schools', to use one phrase (ibid.). The everyday environment is as important as school – and social workers, the experts in everyday life, have particular responsibilities to ensure that care placements and schools are integrated for looked after young people. It is they who join together the practical aspects of living with the relational and the theoretical (ibid.: 9).

The patchy record of corporate parenting

Only 6 per cent of care leavers are in higher education at 19 (the same as 2005), compared to roughly 30 per cent of young people nationally. The proportion of care leavers obtaining five good GCSEs (A–C) is still vastly smaller than for the age group as a whole (Jackson and Cameron 2014; HM Inspectorate of Prisons 2011; Centre for Social Justice 2014).

Twenty per cent of young homeless people were previously in care. Forty-five per cent of girls and young women in prison and 24 per cent of the adult prison population have been in care. As Jackson and Cameron (2014: 26) say, 'Incarceration is the ultimate form of social exclusion.' Poor outcomes continue to roil the social fabric of communities in which care leavers settle. In 2012 some 36 per cent of care leavers were not in education, employment or training (nearly equal to the 38 per cent leaving young offender institutions who are NEET). Seventy per cent of sex workers have been in care. Over 20 per cent of care leavers have drug problems and nearly 40 per cent have mental health difficulties. A high proportion of those leaving care are transferred directly on to the benefit system.

Stein (2012) has roughly divided care leavers into three main groups defined by outcomes: (i) 'Moving on' – the minority who make the transition to adulthood successfully; (ii) 'Surviving' – those who manage to live independently but with many problems and reliant on professional help (although often in conflict with that help); (iii) 'Struggling' – those that have left care before 18 and are poorly prepared to meet the many demands of adult life. For this group, state care fails to prevent exclusion passing from one generation to another (Feinstein et al. 2008). They experience difficulty in maintaining accommodation and become isolated with physical and mental health problems. They are at risk of addiction, sexual exploitation, unplanned pregnancies and criminal activity. Therapeutic engagement, Stein concludes from his research, to deal with their powerful emotions arising from their family troubles, is generally inadequate.

In assisting care leavers to negotiate the transition to adulthood the practitioner has the responsibility to organise support in a number of domains including accommodation, life skills, education, career paths, social networks and relationships, and identity formation. In general those care leavers that have the greatest difficulty have also had the most damaging family experiences before entering care. For them, accommodation may involve initial moves to transitional forms of housing such as hostels, lodgings or staying with friends, which are often followed up by moves to independent tenancies in the public, voluntary or private sectors.

The Children (Leaving Care) Act 2000 imposed duties on local authorities in relation to young people who had been looked after by them: every eligible young person when they turned 16 was to have a clear pathway plan mapping out a route to their independence for which local authorities must provide the personal and practical support. From that point on there was some improvement in the legal framework for supporting care leavers across the four countries of the UK compared with the rest of Western Europe (Stein 2014). But fifteen and more years on, the record on care leavers remains patchy. In an effort to improve the circumstances for care leavers, amendments to the Children Act 1989, the Children and Young Persons Act 2008 and Transition guidance (2014) created a 'staying put' framework to be delivered by the local authority. Acknowledging that the transition to adulthood can be prolonged and turbulent, young people in care may remain in foster placement until the age of 21 (ibid.). Yet despite these moves, Ofsted inspections found that two-thirds of schemes still required improvement or were inadequate (National Audit Office 2015).

Practical support is provided to a care leaver in moving to new accommodation that can be deemed 'sufficient', including an allowance to help furnish and settle into their new home. That package includes out of hours support and the opportunity to be looked after again when under age 18. Special guardianship orders are available for extended family and friends placements.

The Scottish government goes further, recently providing increased support for *all* care leavers – allowing them to stay in care until 21 whether or not they remain in education, and to receive support until age 26.

REFLECT AND DECIDE: WHAT SOCIAL WORKERS SHOULD BE ASKING THEMSELVES REGARDING A CARE LEAVER

Is there enough focus on the young person's pathway plan to ensure that it is of high quality and written in a way that suits the young person and includes their aspirations, pictures, messages? Care leavers often feel their pathway plans are written to meet the local authority's own requirements and not theirs.

Is there sufficient focus on the standard of accommodation for the young person? Has Schedule 2 of the Care Leavers (England) Regulations 2010 been taken into account?

Does the young person have readily available access to information about their care leaver entitlements including the setting up home allowance?

Is the social worker ensuring that the young person has a network of support so that they do not feel alone and experience loneliness?

(adapted from the Care Leavers in England Data Pack; DfE 2012)

TABLE 5.1   Statutory framework for care leavers

Age 16	At least three months before their 16th birthday the young person in care must be given a personal adviser to take over the role of social worker and develop a pathway plan setting out where they will live and what further education or employment they will embark on.
Age 16–18	The young person may leave care but that decision must be signed off by the director of children's services; the local authority must continue to provide assistance for accommodation and living costs; the care leaver retains her or his personal adviser.
Age 18–21	On their 18th birthday the young person ceases to be looked after. The local authority must have developed a pathway plan, maintain contact through a personal adviser, and provide assistance towards education- and/or employment-related costs. Housing costs are usually met through housing benefit unless the care leaver is in further or higher education in which case local authority support continues until the age of 25.

Finding settled accommodation

Despite new regulations, difficulties for care leavers abound. Their major concern revolves around housing – worry over finding suitable and safe accommodation, wondering whether they will manage to live alone, fear of being made homeless. Many care leavers are placed in unsuitable private tenancies. These are often the first tenancy held by a young person – compounded by abrupt changes of location, especially for those who are placed in care out of borough who then move back to a home area once out of care where they may or may not be eligible for priority housing with the new authority (Barnardo's 2014a). Indeed roughly one-third of young people with care backgrounds experience homelessness* at some stage between 6 and 24 months after leaving care (Stein 2010).

While suitable housing is a source of stability and a platform for other youth outcomes, a recent compilation of experiences highlights the missteps by practitioners in settling care leavers (Stein 2010). Care leavers' own view of safe and settled accommodation includes non-housing elements that are within the control of the practitioner:

- having a choice *when* to leave care
- being adequately prepared for leaving care

*Homelessness in this context includes 'sofa surfing' (short stays with family, friends or acquaintances, usually sleeping in a room other than a bedroom), staying at homeless hostels, refuges, or sleeping rough, and periods in B&B accommodation.

- having a choice as to their accommodation and feeling safe in it
- having practical and personal support, including support from family, friends and former carers
- having financial backing
- being able to participate in arranging the services that affect them.

(Stein 2010)

CASE STUDY: A CARE LEAVER'S EXPERIENCE OF 'SUITABLE ACCOMMODATION'

Well, at that time I was 16, so I didn't really know what I wanted. But at that time we have two semi-independent flats about the children's home. So you go through them and then you get your own flat. That's how it is for so many people, so that's what we thought was going to happen. Then one day they said to me that they were moving me to [another area]. So I thought, cool. They moved me to [what] I thought was a children's home. I asked them what [it] was and they said it was a semi-independent. I didn't know anything about this place, they just dumped me there and said this is your place now.

(Barnardo's 2014a)

Resilience in care leavers

If some disadvantaged young people show resilience in coping with the difficulties in leaving care it is logical to ask whether it is possible to promote resilience through various interventions with young people who might otherwise not have it. Gilligan (2008) concluded that developing resilience requires comprehensive services across the young person's life in care and after care that allow for the same gradual, extended transition that young people in general have. There are recognised elements in how to do this: stability of in-care placement, helping the young person develop a positive view of themselves, preparation for living on their own, assistance in connecting to educational institutions, extended support after care (ibid.). Resilience understood this way shifts from an inner quality within the young person that triumphs over adversity to something that is produced through an interaction between individual development and social environment. Resilience in this sense is a quality that draws on services – and needs accessible services – and the personal relationships with practitioners and landlord; it is located within relationships and not dependent on the individual care leaver's personal make-up.

Education and leaving care outcomes

Every year around 10,000 16–18-year-olds leave foster or residential care in England. Some return home, many move on to start independent lives. Low educational attainment makes this transition difficult. While modestly improving year on year in key stages 2 and 3, educational attainment of care leavers is falling at key stage 4. As of

March 2014, at key stage 4, 15 per cent of looked after children achieved five or more GCSEs at grade A*–C including English and mathematics, compared with 58 per cent for the country as a whole, an attainment gap of 43 percentage points (Department for Education 2012b, 2015).

Social workers, with little understanding of the tempo and requirements of secondary education, plan placements that are often unintentionally disruptive, with looked after children spending a considerable portion of time out of education. They focus on emotional support but pay less attention to acquiring skills and knowledge and building lasting friendships. Equally schools and teachers have limited knowledge of the care system and the complexities around taking a child or young person into care, and finding a suitable placement.

All the evidence suggests that education should be at the centre of a care placement. Stability of the placement relates to the stability of the schooling with relationship to teachers and peers. This means paying attention to the young person's education in selection and training of foster carers, with checks on their knowledge of the educational system, and their ability to help young people with homework and to guide them along their educational pathway. In residential care the same principle applies: education should always be considered in reviews and discussed at meetings with young people.

CASE STUDY: FINAN

Finan, 22, who arrived in the UK from Eritrea at age 16, thought he was poorly advised by his leaving care team. He spent four years in a sixth form college acquiring GCSEs but also other lower-level qualifications which he did not need in order to attend university.

> I mean I should [have] qualified by now, but for me I didn't get the right information, it's kind of complicated, a bit wasted . . . I should have been studying in college [on a two year access course] and after gone to uni. That was my plan.
>
> (Huari and Cameron 2014: 99)

Multi-agency partnerships

The looked after young person is 'corporately' parented – that is, the local authority itself, linked to other agencies, local and national, such as the NHS, stands in for the work of upbringing that parents would do. One can immediately see the difficulties for organisations in filling this role. It is divided among carers (foster or residential), draws on various budgets and funding streams (including benefits), and calls on a number of different professionals – children's social workers (who may have the inclination to prioritise care arrangements over education), leaving care teams, teachers or out of school private tutors, school administrators and virtual head teachers. Professionals change posts, they go on holiday, they fall sick – only one of the many sources of discontinuity that will hamper the plan around the care leaver whether in regard to education or accommodation.

Closer multi-agency working across the care system is the only means to surmount these difficulties, bringing together careers advice, welfare benefits and legal advice, health and mental health support and education support workers or mentors. In one area that Huari and Cameron (2014) examined they found three teams with overlapping responsibilities for leaving care: a leaving care team for those aged 16–24, a long-term children and young persons' team for those in care over age 7, and a looked after children health and education services team that aimed to raise aspirations and develop agency. Leaving care is long-term and begins when the child is first looked after. Avoiding alienation from education, addressing low levels of numeracy and literacy, meeting issues of self-confidence and personal efficacy begins at key stages 1, 2 and 3 with extra tuition and an array of other supports and resources. Ball and Vincent distinguish between 'cold knowledge' – information from reference books, printed sources or the internet – and 'hot knowledge' – sources of information from people who know the education options, have informed contacts and personal experience. Social workers do not often come into this second category (1998: 99).

KEY POINTS

❑   The transition to adulthood is a prolonged time of trial and error; public resources, rites of passage, guidance from trusted adults to help adolescents navigate through it are in short supply. For excluded youth the burden of individual risk is highest.

❑   Individual relationships with practitioners are all-important. Evidence tells us that mentoring, reparative and social pedagogic relationships have lasting effects on the disaffected adolescent in their progress to adulthood.

❑   Anti-social behaviour is defined and responded to locally, providing room for restorative justice approaches.

❑   The extent of child sexual exploitation points up the limitations of an individual, forensic approach to dealing with child abuse. To counter it requires understanding neighbourhood networks and mapping hot spots.

❑   Despite fifteen years and more since the Leaving Care Act 2000 was implemented, progress in improving outcomes for care leavers has been slow. Improved educational attainment and securing settled accommodation are the twin pillars for the successful transition to independence.

KEY READING

Claire Cameron, Graham Connelly and Sonia Jackson, *Educating Children and Young People in Care: Learning Placements and Caring Schools* (Jessica Kingsley Publishers, 2015). This team of authors, and Jackson in particular, have been focusing for a long time on how poorly children and young people are educated once they are in care. Moving on from the deficits they argue passionately for bringing the ethos of education and care together in both care and school settings.

Gerald Patterson, *Anti-social Boys* (Catania Publishing, 1992). Patterson explains clearly how the seeds of anti-social behaviour can be sown early on through patterns of 'coercive parenting'. His work is one of the chief influences behind parent training schemes.

Nick Luxmore, *Working with Anger and Young People* (Jessica Kingsley Publishers, 2006). Luxmore reports from the street level with wide experience of working directly with young people – and draws on his years of conversations with young people, both troubled and untroubled.

Cordelia Fine, *Delusions of Gender* (Icon Books, 2012). A revanchist gender stereotyping is underway in Britain – with domestic violence, sexual exploitation and internet threats of harm and sadism at its cutting edge. Fine's book is a science-based reply to some of the justifications for the 'softer' end of this oppression, including the neuroscience argument that 'girls will be girls and boys will be boys'.

CHAPTER 6

SOCIAL CARE AND EXCLUDED ADULTS

THIS CHAPTER COVERS

- The extent of social exclusion among adults: chronic ill health, frailty in old age and disability.

- Exclusion and the social care system: personalisation and individual budgets.

- Adults of working age, work capability assessments and personal resilience.

- Neighbourhood-based solutions to minimise the effects of dementia and loneliness.

SOCIAL EXCLUSION AMONG ADULTS

This chapter deals with the various ways adults are excluded. They may be in poverty from insufficient income or barriers to their entry into the labour market. They may suffer ill health and the consequences of health inequalities. They can be alienated from their own care planning, without influence over decisions and unaware of their rights. Or they may be isolated simply through poorly performing or non-existent networks or other features of the environment such as poor housing or a menacing atmosphere in public places. The main features of adult exclusion are:

- *Poverty* in old age is at its lowest on record largely because pensions have been uprated regularly, a greater than ever percentage of older people own their own homes, and benefits specific to older people, such as the winter heating allowance, have been protected regardless of income level. On the other hand, around 20 per cent of pensioners still live in relative poverty, which particularly curtails their social connections such as seeing friends and family regularly or going on a holiday, while 10 per cent are materially deprived (Kotecha and Coutinho n.d.).

- *Withdrawal of services*: the number of people receiving publicly commissioned adult social care services fell by one-quarter between 2009/10 and 2013/14, from 1.7 million to below 1.3 million. Care at home and other community-based services were hit especially hard, resulting in an average 8 per cent reduction in the number of users each year. Overall by 2013/14, 17.4 per cent less was being spent on services for older people. By contrast, the number of people aged 65 and over increased by 10.1 per cent over the same period, including an 8.6 per cent increase in the population aged 85 or over (Burchardt *et al.* 2015).
- *Poverty* among working-age adults is at its highest. This is in part because of cuts in tax credits that provide financial support for in-work parents and in part because wages only just returned to pre-crisis levels in 2014. In 2012/13 nearly half of adults in poverty, well over 3.2 million, were in households where *all* adults work – virtually the same number as in workless families. When households where at least one adult was working were included, that number doubled: a total of 6.6 million people in 'working families' were living in poverty – the same as the number of people who were out of work (MacInnes *et al.* 2014: 30). In short, there was no difference in numbers between those experiencing 'in work' poverty and 'out of work' poverty.

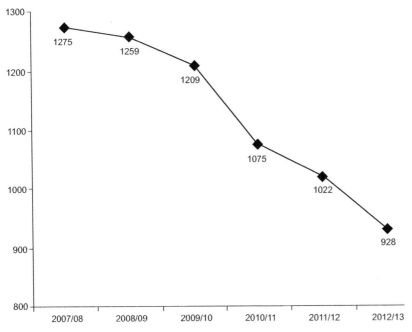

FIGURE 6.1   Reduction in social care recipients, England (000s) (reproduced with permission from the Care and Support Alliance)

- By 2013 *unemployment* among men and women between 20 and 24 had reached 12 per cent (Hills 2015). In 2012–13 median income for those in their twenties and thirties was 18 per cent lower after housing costs than five years before (ibid.: 4). The median income for Black adults fell by more than any other group: by 12.3 per cent after housing costs, and for the poorest Black adults by 22 per cent.
- *Bangladeshi men* had the lowest full-time median hourly wage – £10.00 – and the lowest full-time employment rate, just 20 per cent in 2013 (ibid.: 5).
- The number of *users* drawing on services among working-age adults with mental health problems dropped by 37 per cent and the number of physically disabled users aged 65 or over fell by 32 per cent (Burchardt *et al.* 2015).

SOCIAL CARE AND EXCLUSION

In the 1990s, following implementation of the NHS and Community Care Act, 'care' in the community became synonymous with care at home, and in practice relied on informal care from families to look after those in need rather than placing individual need in the context of community networks and resources (Barr *et al.* 1997). The late Gerald Smale (Smale *et al.* 1993, 2000), who was both prescient and ignored in his time by mainstream practice, urged social workers to support carers through neighbourhood work and strengthened social networks. Concepts such as negotiation and partnership, collaboration with community groups and the value of local knowledge all figure prominently in his thinking, so that his work is still fresh and relevant today (Smale *et al.* 2000).

When social care practice relies on informal carers from within the family, or on low-paid staff, women predominantly shoulder the main burden and responsibility for providing that care. The argument made by feminists is that caring is essentially a gendered activity and that community care policies rely on this fact but do not acknowledge it. To refer only to 'carers', without also specifying the fact that the preponderance of caring is carried out by women, hides the exploitation on which the policy is based and without which it could not succeed. Ungendered references to 'carers' suggest that who carries out caring tasks is not important and at the same time underwrite the assumption that women will take up these tasks as a matter of course.

This has the effect of perpetuating the general subordination of women in what dominant social convention considers an informal set of chores that carries little or no value in the labour market. The exploitation, it can be argued, extends also to those who carry out care tasks within the public services such as home carers, district nurses and residential care workers. Because caring carries little public recognition those that perform it may themselves undervalue their own work. Thus the concepts of 'community care' and the now more ubiquitous 'social care' mask the different roles assigned to men and women that need to be clarified in order to build an inclusionary practice around them. If community care is little more than another ideological device to extract unpaid, underpaid and low-prestige labour out of women, then it is an oppressive, exclusionary concept in its own right, exacting a 'care penalty' according to Nancy Folbre (2001).

Social work decision making in adult social care

While the issues of resourcing and hiving off care work to 'family' – mainly women – are perennial, the kind of activity that social workers undertake has changed significantly since the NHS and Community Care Act 1991. Professional roles have been divided and power to command resources diluted; budgets have been dispersed in the now mostly private market. Social workers' discretion in deciding adult care outcomes has become correspondingly narrower. Without the kind of consensus that to some degree has protected social work with children, evident for example in the outcry that forced the Coalition government to back away from plans to privatise child protection services in 2014, adult social care has been opened up to every conceivable initiative and manoeuvre – from the top of government in the form of the NHS and Social Care Act 2013, to entirely local efforts, volunteer, charitable and private – to supply the missing parts of a once unified service. As Malcolm Carey has observed. 'The protected professional term "social work" fits uneasily with such bureaucratic processes which help hold together, administrate and, crucially, gate-keep and ration access to finite services within ever more fragmented systems of social care' (Carey 2014: 7). Carey concludes that one of the main activities of care managers is to refuse to provide a service.

There is an important debate over how much discretion social workers still retain in social care decisions. Ellis acknowledges that areas of discretion exist but concludes that 'the assessment and care management systems both lessen managers' dependency on frontline discretion to deliver desired results and smooth out conflicting interests' (Ellis 2011: 231). Technology enables top-down prescription and enforcement of procedures. The various stages of assessment are defined on-screen. Initial assessments are made over the telephone while the practitioner completes the 'paperwork' on computer; from the outset, early stages of referral and initial assessment are geared toward eligibility criteria. Together this narrows the scope for value-based practice – for example incorporating users' definition of need.

On the other hand there is evidence that practitioners see room for discretion, with a broad range of attitudes to following rules and procedures. Even in rule-saturated organisations, social workers retain significant freedom in their work, and individual practitioner attitudes toward organisational rules are key to understanding how they use that discretion in decision making (Evans 2013). Evans found two different orientations toward policies and procedures among practitioners: those that emphasised procedural rules designed to ensure equal outcomes across the board, and those that emphasised fair outcomes for specific individuals and were willing to bend rules to achieve them. Practitioners in this latter group thought ethical commitment to the individual user took precedence over equality of procedure and that official policies reflected an impoverished conception of need that had to be expanded through professional reinterpretation.

For assessment under the Care Act 2014, the practitioner needs to consider six themes at each stage of the assessment and eligibility process: (i) mental capacity; (ii) advocacy and support of user participation; (iii) impact on the family and carers; (iv) safeguarding; (v) a strengths-based approach; (vi) proportionate and appropriate decisions (DoH 2013, 2014b). These categories centre on the individual and immediate family with no reference to neighbourhood conditions or other elements of the macro environment. The adult outcomes framework, which gives an annual account closely tied to the Care Act, is really an annual rating of service performance and the degree to which users are satisfied, used for benchmarking and comparing local authorities, covering four domains:

- Ensuring quality of life for people with care and support needs.
- Delaying and reducing the need for care and support.
- Ensuring that people have a positive experience of care and support.
- Safeguarding adults whose circumstances make them vulnerable.

CARE ACT 2014

The Care Act 2014 places personalisation on a statutory footing, enshrining in law the principle that each individual should be at the centre of decision making concerning the care service they are to receive. Under the Act local authorities are required to develop strategies for providing information, such as online databases, and advice to help users make sense of social care provision in their area from voluntary, public, health and social care organisations. It further requires local authorities to:

- Carry out an assessment of anyone who appears to need care, regardless of whether or not that person is eligible for state funding.
- Focus assessment on the outcomes the person wants to achieve.
- Involve the person and their carer if appropriate in assessment, providing an independent advocate if needed.
- Establish close collaboration between health and social care through the Better Care Fund planning, and digital links. For the first time the adult social care outcomes framework (ASCOF) will include a measure of whether people experience care that is joined-up and seamless.

The Care Act 2014 and guide to the Act stipulate that to strengthen the local approach to self-assessment commissioners of services have a duty to promote a 'vibrant and responsive market of service providers', to ensure that services reflect the diversity of the population and local needs. To do this means being open to new ways of doing things and 'sharing the endeavour' across commissioners, providers, users and their families.

REFLECT AND DECIDE: NEW WAYS OF CREATING A VIBRANT MARKET IN ADULT SOCIAL CARE

- Map the current market provision.
- Specify what a more diverse market would look like in a particular locality.

- Involve users at the commissioning stage.
- Ensure the market positioning statement addresses diversity.
- Ensure that services are publicised.

(adapted from TLAP – Think Local, Act Personal)

Think through how this 'vibrant market' will take place in the locality in which you work.

Believers in the 'efficient market' and the capacity of users to make rational choices will find much to be enthusiastic about here. Alternatively, focus on markets is accelerating the fragmentation of the service environment, with no clear chain of responsibility or way to enforce rules, no explicit rights for users and no way to seek redress when rules and regulations are breached. Providers will come and go, enter into and pull out of contracts, sell on their user base and perhaps buy others, begin as ethical social enterprises on their way to becoming profit-oriented. Web-based portals for users will become universal and further distance personal communication including for those seeking redress. While local authority and NHS-provided services have long had to meet performance measurements and targets – with their reputation rising and falling as a single 'public sector' – a market system as a whole has no such judgement made on its overall performance. Individual companies and agencies may be held to account if they fail to deliver as promised (although private sector organisations often reveal their shortcomings only after prolonged periods of failure, for example Atos in the field of work capability assessment).

REFLECT AND DECIDE: UNDERSTANDING MARKETS IN SOCIAL CARE

The Care Act envisages churning in the market for care provision.

Markets of any kind will naturally involve a degree of entry and exit of providers and this will be of limited concern where it results in maintained or higher service quality overall. However, it is possible that a succession of market exits may jeopardise the diversity and sustainability of the market. When considering the impact of a market exit on diversity and sustainability it is advisable to segment the local social care market into sub-markets (for example buildings-based and non-buildings-based, or urban and rural settings). By segmenting the market it is easier for a local authority to ensure they are taking a proportionate and efficient approach, with time and resource dedicated to responding to market exits targeted towards those areas of the market which are less sustainable.

(TLAP Commissioning for Market Diversity, www.thinklocalactpersonal.org.uk/co-production-in-commissioning)

Specifically, what personnel in the local authority will undertake to segment the market into 'sub-markets' with the time and knowledge to respond to market exits? How and in what form will local authorities be able to respond to 'less sustainable' areas of provision within the market?

With care increasingly lucrative, market-based care provision is seen as a way of reducing the power of local authorities and meeting the concern that people were being shunted into services that were designed to suit councils. What are the merits of this argument?

CASE STUDY: CONNECT TO SUPPORT

Local authorities across Yorkshire and the Humber have collaborated regionally to develop the Connect to Support platform for adult social care, providing information and advice, assessments and screening, personal budget management, brokerage, care accounts and a transactional e-Marketplace. Connect to Support provides an 'open market' where people can choose and purchase care, or equipment that best suits their needs and identified outcomes, directly. Connect to Support utilises the PCG Care Solutions platform and has been live in local authority areas across the region since 2012. There are currently some 580 provider stores across the Yorkshire and Humber region, containing over 4,500 individually priced products and services that are available to buy online, together with over 10,000 entries for local groups and activities.

PERSONALISATION AND INDEPENDENCE

Oliver (1990) has long argued that professionals and disabled people do not talk about the same thing when discussing independence. The former view it in terms of self-care activities and the skills needed to carry them out. The latter see independence as being able to make decisions about their lives and exercise control over the way those decisions are carried out, not about being able to perform activities for oneself without assistance. Attitudes toward personal safety, dignity and self-respect and use of public money all impact on decisions about independence – how people make choices about support services and how those choices have consequences, not always realised at the time, on their independence in the long term. The question is how can independence be preserved when care arrangements are reliant on others, specifically health and social care practitioners, to carry out care?

Some argue that it is possible to differentiate between 'decisional' and 'executional' autonomy, particularly in work with older people – those who are able to maintain a sense of self and control over decisions but letting other people carry them out (Rabiee 2013: 874). Others would sidestep this debate altogether by arguing that the concept of 'interdependency' based on partnership and a sense of joint responsibility should replace the dispute over dependency and autonomy. This contains its own difficulties in as much as it subsumes a vital principle – independence and autonomy

– into aspirational hopes about partnerships and mutuality (both giving and receiving care) that may or may not be realised in practice. Still others argue that the concept of autonomy must remain unconditional and undiluted as a bulwark against a loss of freedoms, not least that brought about by collapsing services and bewildering pathways through those services that do remain.

Rabiee's research established that the notion of independence is not a fixed concept – but relative, conditional and multi-dimensional. Its meanings varied from person to person. She found that most people associated the *loss* of their independence with being forced into making a particular 'choice' because there were no realistic alternatives, while *independence* was 'being in control, able to do things on your own, freedom of movement when and where you want, self-sufficiency, the confidence to be who you are, financial security, living in your own home' (ibid.: 877). Independence requires reaching a practical balance between doing things for oneself and knowing when to ask for help. Attaining such a balance becomes more complex in the face of new impairments, the rise in the numbers of those with long-term impairment, and a larger ageing population living longer but with long-term health problems.

Personal budgets

The introduction of personal budgets (PB), as the centre piece of personalisation, under the Putting People First programme, was intended to improve on the earlier system of direct payments (DoH 2010). They are now obligatory for all adult social care users, backed up by a new sector-wide partnership, Think Local, Act Personal, which offers resources, tools and support for introducing personal budgets (www.thinklocalact personal.org.uk) – with funding determined by an assessment of the person's financial contribution to the costs of support.

The stated aim of personal budgets is to give people more control over the resources for their care and support, underpinned by the proposition that individuals themselves are in the best position to identify the kinds of support they need and enabling them to draw on their own social networks as well as professional contacts. Personal budgets can be in the form of dedicated funding or a service – or a combination of both. People may plan and manage their own support if they want to, knowing the level of resources available to them. A range of personnel – social workers, social care managers, but also generic care planners or relatives or friends – support the planning process through which individuals' priorities and aims are formulated. A senior manager signs off the plan while at the same time considering risks and possible safeguarding issues.

With personal budgets the sense of autonomy and control comes at a price. As Smale *et al.* (1993: 6) long ago noted:

> Being a customer with money in your pocket is not an insurance against powerlessness. It is difficult for users to make real choices when their past experience of using social services is limited. There is always the tendency for 'people to want what they know rather than know what they want'.

Glendinning *et al.* (2008) argued that those in need of social care may be unwilling or unable to undertake the search for information on the service that would suit them best. Moreover, where needs are specialised, or in areas where few services are available in the first place, the principles of personalisation are difficult to carry out. Those that lack both the resources and the knowledge required to make a system of personal budgets function smoothly, will be the casualties in an arrangement that places more responsibility on individuals, families and carers and less on central or local authorities for optimising social care (Glendinning *et al.* 2008).

Evaluations of personal budgets suggest that only modest improvements in adult care outcomes have been achieved. Netten and colleagues undertook substantial random controlled trials, following a group of users with individual budgets and a group without. On the basis of quality of life measures at six months they found no statistically significant differences between the PB and comparison groups. They did find however that the PB group reported a greater *feeling* of control over their daily lives compared with the non-PB group (48 to 41 per cent) – especially among those with a learning disability. The process around PBs with the linked supported planning marked an important gain in users' sense of 'agency' – the control and capacity to achieve objectives on their own initiative. Netten *et al.* also found that quality of life for people with mental health problems was higher in the PB group than the non-PB group. Older people, however, within the PB group reported significantly *lower* wellbeing than the comparison group (Netten *et al.* 2012: 1564).

The impact of PBs, then, depends on the user group. Those adults with mental health difficulties were especially receptive and showed improved outcomes. There were more limited gains in outcomes for adults with learning disability – though social workers needed to carry an advocacy role to realise those outcomes. Older people, on the other hand, suffered a negative impact on psychological wellbeing. Older people in the PB group did not feel in greater control but experienced higher levels of anxiety during the planning and support phase. To elicit opinions of users the researchers at some points had to use proxies, that is get opinions of others who were close to the individuals and knowledgeable about their wishes and hopes. When the views stated by proxies were excluded, differences between the PB and non-PB groups became statistically insignificant. Essentially the findings confirmed an earlier round of PB evaluations of 2005–7, giving some stability to those findings over time (Jacobs *et al.* 2013).

Personal budgets and adult social care practice

Such evaluations highlight the complexities for practitioners and adult care coordinators implementing PBs within an inclusionary practice. One study found that on most measures there were no differences in working patterns between care managers with and those without PB holders on their caseload. However, the results do show that – contrary to expectations – more time was spent assessing needs, and that more time generally was required for support planning activities.

There is also some risk in relation to older people with dementia, a group that suffers high rates of financial abuse and exploitation. While the Mental Capacity Act of 2005 offered safeguards when an individual lacks capacity, those who are mildly confused, less vigilant or otherwise vulnerable were not so protected. While there are powers available to the police, the Court of Protection and the Benefits Agency to block the unsuitable and unscrupulous from having influence over a personal budget, in general social workers need to be alert to signs of financial abuse, with regular financial reviews that would highlight inconsistencies in spending (Manthorpe and Samsi 2013).

Moreover, personal budgets when fully rolled out could threaten collective models of social care. For example, an older person living in a housing with care scheme may not choose to spend their individual budget with the scheme's care provider, thus undermining the funding for this core service – a service from which all the residents in the scheme benefit because of the peace of mind that an *in situ* carer on the premises provides (Blood 2013). This is the classic 'free-rider' dilemma: an individual benefits from an asset that others are paying for – and by not contributing thereby undermining the provision of that asset.

REFLECT AND DECIDE: THE IMPACT OF PERSONAL BUDGETS ON SERVICES

if no one tells you what the budget is or what you can do and what – how, you know what I mean, and if that's in the budget to cover . . . no one gives you the information. If you ask for it, they say, 'We don't know'.

(Rabiee and Glendinning 2014: 7)

I don't like complaining. And I won't complain unless I have to complain . . . I'll put up with it. I'm not, you know – I don't want to cause any trouble, like, you know . . . But it sometimes – it annoys my husband sometimes, but it can't be helped . . . I just go with the flow. It makes it easier, makes it simpler.

(ibid.: 8)

What actions should the practitioner take in response to such statements from users? What practice guidelines would need to be drawn up to ensure there is a balance between individual rights to an individual budget and collective arrangements for social care – that the former would not undermine the latter?

While many local authorities begin the PB process with a self-assessment questionnaire, it is difficult to distinguish those users that can complete this knowledgeably and confidently and those that require supported self-assessment or practitioner-completed assessment – albeit still 'person centred' (SCIE 2014). There are differences too among individual practitioners. Some have little difficulty in leaving the person to complete their own self-assessment questionnaire, while others want to remain involved. There is a wider tendency to assume that older people are less able to undertake self-assessment, making the process more time-consuming, especially for older people's teams accustomed to faster handling of assessments (ibid.). Approximately two-thirds have their PBs managed by their council and they are largely used to purchase council-commissioned services. In a recent survey only two of eighteen interviewees knew they had a budget allocated to them, or who to contact about funding flexibility, for example when extra care visits were required following discharge from hospital (Rabiee and Glendinning 2014).

PERSONAL BUDGETS – GOOD PRACTICE POINTS

- Importance of clear, understandable information about what a personal budget is, how it can be used and what is involved in holding one.
- Time spent discussing personal budgets with the holder's social worker, community psychiatric nurse, support provider organisation (SPO) or peer/user organisation support worker is more helpful than written information.
- Clear basic guidance on 'using your personal budget' that explains the link between expenditure and the support plan. A named member of staff (or team), familiar with the personal budget holder's circumstances.
- Guidance (and training) for local authority, mental health trust and SPO staff on the use of personal budgets and scope for team managers to approve special requests.
- Maximising user control regardless of how the PB is managed.

There are important steps for organisations tackling exclusion to take in relation to personal budgets. These include: (i) the opportunity to exchange ideas with other agencies about how they use personal budgets; (ii) outreach to marginalised communities through trusted networks; (iii) introducing guidelines and procedures for linking risk assessment – particularly financial exploitation – to support planning; (iv) widening service provisions to enable greater and more attractive choices. There are also measures to prevent the PB process becoming too complex for the user: for example, creating a stable and trusting relationship between user (the PB holder) and practitioner by giving staff training, supervision support and the time to work through the decisions that the user has to make. It also helps to devolve authority to local teams, allowing practitioners to develop their process most effectively (SCIE 2014).

The greater argument over the nature of personalisation discourse will continue. The issue is whether it is a step toward social citizenship, allowing previously excluded users to enjoy the full benefits of society, or whether it takes consumerist, not professional, ideals into social care, importing as well all of the inequalities of markets, with consumers reliant on diminishing funding from government as their source of purchasing power (Lymbery 2014).

ADULTS WITH DISABILITY

People with disability articulated the experience of exclusion long before it became a concept in social policy. Their discussion and practitioners' responses contribute extensively to our current understanding of exclusion as a social process – from the labour market, to shopping mobility, to simple access to buildings and across city streets. Generally, social work in the past based its practice towards people with disability on the basis of 'individual pathology' and meeting individual needs (disability in the Children Act 1989 automatically renders a child 'in need'). Disability was defined as a set of deficits and needs, and practitioners approached disabled people and their families holding attitudes that linked disability with dependency and care. For decades services were segregated through special schools, adult training centres, residential establishments and long-stay hospitals. Separate leisure facilities are still common with clubs and special holidays still undertaken in groups.

This legacy of segregation underpinned a depth of discriminatory attitudes in society at large based on a toxic mix of distaste, distance, pity and condescension. Disabled people felt the full force of multi-layered exclusion: low income through inadequate benefits, exclusion from the labour market, exclusion from cultural and intellectual activity, and disrupted social networks. They also faced a variety of threats to their very existence. One threat came from legal judgments that a potentially disabled foetus can be aborted, while others feared that court-sanctioned euthanasia of those in a 'vegetative state' was the start of a slippery slope that could extend to other disabling conditions. The latter raised within disabled groups the explicit memory of the National Socialist programme in Germany in the 1930s that undertook the first mass euthanasia of disabled people (Burleigh 1994).

Largely through persistent advocacy and argument, dedicated activity and civic protest, disabled people have shaped and communicated a positive idea of disability. The social model focuses on how social attitudes have excluded people with impairments. It is society and not the disabled person that has failed to adjust. In this view disabled people do not need a mobility allowance but a transport system that eliminates the barriers to people with impaired mobility. The way homes are constructed does not cater for physical capabilities; the world of work is geared to maximising profit from the able-bodied (Oliver and Sapey 2006). In essence the social model lays out a political strategy – better to pursue barrier removal and social change than seek rehabilitation and cure.

THE SOCIAL MODEL

In our view, it is society which disables physically impaired people. Disability is something imposed on top of our impairments by the way we are unnecessarily isolated and excluded from full participation in society. To understand this it is necessary to grasp the distinction between the physical impairment and the social situation, called 'disability', of people with such an impairment. Disability [is] the disadvantage or restriction of activity caused by a contemporary social organisation which takes no or little account of people who have physical impairments and thus excludes them from the mainstream of social activities.

(from a statement by the Union of the Physically Impaired Against Segregation, 1976, quoted in Oliver and Sapey 2006: 22)

Shakespeare has argued that the very success of the social model is now its main weakness – 'a sacred cow, an ideology which could not easily be challenged' (Shakespeare and Watson 2002: 12). Through it organisations and policies are judged quickly: have they used the term 'disabled people' (social model) or did they use 'people with disabilities' (medical model)? Did they focus on barrier removal or on medical intervention and rehabilitation? To some extent this rigid dichotomy became a litmus test for disability activists and discouraged public discussion about impairments and their impact on the person's functioning. This, according to Shakespeare, is an unsustainable distinction: where does impairment end and disability start? After all, achieving a 'barrier free' environment is impossible – removing barriers for one kind of disability may mean creating a barrier for others. He adopts what he calls a materialist analysis of disability, arguing that impairment itself is a social phenomenon, and talking about impairment and how it links to 'embodiment' – being human – rather than focusing exclusively on social barriers to those with impairment, is a legitimate goal for the disability movement (ibid.: 2002).

Work capability assessment

The employment rate of working-age people with disability was 46 per cent as of 2012. While that percentage had improved by 10 per cent between 1998 and 2008, it had remained flat since then – a full 30 per cent lower than that of working-age non-disabled people, by far the lowest of all the major groups of excluded adults. Disabled people consistently report that they would like to work, but regardless of qualifications held – whether degree, A levels, GCSEs or none – the proportion of people with a disability who want to work but remain without work is much greater than those without a disability (Palmer et al. 2008: 71). Nineteen per cent of working-age disabled people hold no formal qualifications, compared to 6.5 per cent of non-disabled people. Fifteen per cent of working-age disabled people hold a degree-level qualification as opposed to 28 per cent of non-disabled (DWP 2014).

When work capability assessment (WCA) replaced personal capability assessment, which had determined eligibility for incapacity benefit, it marked a shift toward a functional assessment – what a person can physically and cognitively do – as opposed to a condition-based approach. WCA aims to find out two things: whether the claimant has a limited capability for work *and* whether that claimant has a limited capability to undertake work-related activity. The two are not the same. The first test decides whether the claimant can remain on Employment Support Allowance (ESA). It is based on points relating to physical, mental and cognitive activities (called 'descriptors') that the person may or may not be able to carry out. If the claimant has sufficient points from across these various activities – that is, unable to carry them out – she or he 'passes' the test and remains on ESA. The second test decides whether the claimant is able to undertake work-related activity, again based on a range of tasks that they may or may not be able to do. If they cannot achieve a certain number of these activities they are placed in the Support Group; if they can, they are placed in the work-related activity group for skills training and writing job applications. Failure to meet these conditions can lead to the ESA benefit being sanctioned. (For the descriptors see *A Guide to Employment and Support Allowance – The Work Capability Assessment*, ESA214.)

The new suite of work-oriented benefits can present uncomfortable questions for a practitioner working with people with long-term health conditions or disability. The benefits system applies time limits and tasks that may be difficult to complete. Fear of sanctions, pressure to find work that may be beyond the capacity of the individual, and anxiety over the future are part of the process. To deliver back-to-work support, government depends on a range of public, private and voluntary sector providers. Helping those in the transition from benefit to work, then, depends on effective joint working with local employment services to provide integrated support – and this may or may not be present. For the social worker, full exploration with the user in negotiating the consequences of such a system becomes an overriding objective.

Various groups of adult users have been adversely caught up in the WCA process. The Litchfield review (2014), for example, found widespread difficulties in actually assessing capability of those with mental health problems, in part because diagnostic labels are unhelpful in understanding the impact of the condition on functional capacity. It discovered that: (i) those with mental health problems found answering the questions on the ESA50 questionnaire too difficult; and (ii) health care professionals often did not listen carefully and placed an undue focus on physical conditions when mental health was the prime cause of incapacity.

The review also found difficulties for ex-offenders released from prison with incapacities that predated their sentence. A high proportion of prisoners – more than 70 per cent by some estimates – have two or more mental health disorders, with those with a learning disability perhaps between 5 and 10 per cent. Eligibility for ESA stops when an individual goes to prison, unlike when going to hospital. Those in prison for less than six weeks and receiving contribution-based ESA can ask for their benefit to resume once they are released. But those who are in prison for more than six weeks, and all of those in receipt of income-related ESA, have to make a new claim for ESA when they are released. The claim is processed as normal and the expectation is that a WCA will be undertaken regardless of the reassessment period under a previous claim. Prisoners did not understand why they had to submit a new application when they were already in the Support Group with a long-term award and with a date for a reassessment that was already scheduled long after their release (ibid.).

The private assessment firm originally under contract to the DWP, Atos, was widely regarded as running tests that were crude and inhumane, particularly in relation to disabled people. It was replaced in March 2015 by Maximus – another private contractor – rather than bringing the work back inside the DWP. Determined to run a better system, it hired disability advocates, including from Disability Rights UK, to train those carrying out assessments. Problems of fairness persist: removal of legal aid funding for advice on welfare rights as well as continuing reduction in local authority spending on advice services greatly reduced the support for claimants in challenging benefit decisions. A system of 'Mandatory Reconsideration' on all decisions was introduced in October 2013, an adjudication process that denies an appeal to an independent tribunal *until* the claimant has been phoned at home twice and is compelled to discuss their case with a DWP official on their own without legal or advice support. Taken together they have significantly reduced the number of appeals on assessments from 50,000 in July 2013 to 8,775 in March 2014 (Siddique 2014).

CASE STUDY: TIM SALTER

Tim suffered from mental health problems, among them agoraphobia – fear of open space. He had attempted suicide in 1989, an attempt that left him partially sighted. He was assessed by Atos as to whether he was fit for work but when he told the health care professionals that he sometimes felt suicidal his statement was interpreted as *not* to be 'a declaration of an intention to attempt suicide'. He was deemed fit for work in 2012 and when he did not pursue work his incapacity benefit was cut. In September 2013 he committed suicide. His sister found his body – and also found no food in the house, no money in his bank account and in the dustbin a letter from his housing association threatening him with eviction.

(Karen McVeigh, 'Bereaved sister calls on DWP . . .', *Guardian*, 12 January 2015)

Familiarity with the lengthy WCA questionnaire is a good starting point in offering sustained support for the claimant. WCA is based on a rehabilitative, medical model. Linked to the contravention of the principles of natural justice that the removal of benefits entails, noted in Chapter 3, the WCA is a lopsided process in which the benefit regulators hold all the cards.

From this position of powerlessness of individual claimants practical issues arise. The disabled person and social worker jointly may consider how and in what ways a person is 'work capable'. This could include looking at how training centres might be used to enhance particular skills or how personal budgets could allow users to purchase their own training or equipment in preparation for employment. Or it could include using a 'permitted work opportunity' through which an ESA claimant can take on limited work while still receiving ESA – especially if this can be shown to facilitate take-up of more sustained work later. Other partners such as local user and advocacy groups, local rehabilitation providers, supported employment agencies, or local education authorities could help, as could housing, transport and economic regeneration.

Supported employment

People with learning disability have regularly voiced their aspiration to have a job, yet during the 1990s the daily routine for most was days spent in day centres, training centres or sheltered workshops, segregated from their non-disabled peers and earning negligible wages. The concept of supported employment has partially supplanted the day centre model: a person with learning disability is helped by a supported employment agency in job coaching, job finding, providing internships or work experience that matches their skills and interests. The case is in part economic – a recent Scope report highlights the saving to the public purse and the reduction of poverty among disabled people (Scope 2015). The people who provide support tend to have a variety of job titles such as job coaches, employment advisers, employment consultants and employment support officers. They help develop a vocational profile by identifying skills and work preferences; they also link with would-be employers and develop specific jobs for individuals, offering enough assistance but not undermining independence and growth of skills. Jobcentre Plus staff, Disability Employment Advisors, Care Managers, schools and colleges are often a key referral route into supported employment. Individuals can also self-refer. A person's line manager and colleagues in the workplace can also provide support; they are sometimes called 'natural supports'.

Access to supported employment remains difficult. The benefit system brings difficulties through its lack of familiarity with the concept. As supported employment is not a local authority requirement, programmes are vulnerable to expenditure cuts, with a number of programmes receiving reduced funding or closing altogether (BASE 2014). While the Work Programme supports unemployed disabled people to return to work, only 5 per cent on ESA find a job through it – the number of learning disabled people is minuscule as the Work Programme does not target those with significant needs.

OLD AGE AND SOCIAL EXCLUSION

Old age is described by Erik Erikson as beginning at that point where a person has already reached the peak of their accomplishments, or if not is facing stagnation and self-absorption. The older person is in a transition to that final stage in which all prior stages are integrated with a sense of validity and appreciation, or if not falling into despair, regret and fear (Erikson 1965). Understanding how old age is socially constructed is an important first step in seeing the process whereby older people are excluded through ageism. The social conventions produce 'invisibility' which presumes a lack of sexual interest, an array of physical weaknesses and the inability to work. Yet, as Bill Bytheway reminds us, 'old age' has no real scientific basis since there is no clearly identifiable set of physical changes that marks a person's entry into old age at a given point in time (Bytheway 1995). Physiologically the body changes and is less accomplished in different ways throughout life, but often with compensating strengths developing at the same time.

Older people experience multiple forms of exclusion – through social isolation, reduced services, and barriers to participating in neighbourhood life (Scharf et al. 2005). Exclusionary forces gather pace as a person grows older: the older person may be out of the job market or have a precarious hold on it; friends die, children grow up, income falls off after retirement. While there is growing evidence that personal networks have a protective effect on health and wellbeing at all ages, as they erode with ageing, so that effect wears off (Sluzki 2000). The life course of the older individual affects network strength that thins out and becomes less responsive.

More than half of all people aged 75 and over in the UK live alone. Age UK estimates that over 1 million people say they are often, or always lonely, while some 180,000 of those over 65 say they have gone for a week without speaking to friends, neighbours or family (Age UK n.d.). Social and economic changes have also had an impact. Local services – district nursing, meals on wheels, in-home social care, public transport – have been pared back, while post offices, libraries, shops and pubs have closed in localities across Britain.

Older people with high support needs

Many older people with high support needs receive little from public services: they look after themselves with help from family, friends and neighbours. Some 800,000 of the 2 million older people with high needs receive no support from public services or private care agencies (Age UK 2012). The oldest generations are also now more diverse in terms of ethnicity, faith and sexual orientation; social identity and personal identity are interwoven with greater variations in family arrangements, attitudes to gender, and divorce. For those receiving care it is perhaps understandable that providers place a priority on physical care and protection from risk. However the most important outcomes that older people themselves seek, after personal comfort, are to do with participation in social networks and neighbourhood affairs linked closely to their sense of independence (Netten *et al.* 2006; Carrier 2005).

To understand the wishes of older people takes additional practitioner time as problems with memory, cognitive difficulties, depression or physical incapacities affect expression. 'Unlocking the whole person', in Blood's memorable phrase, that is, responding to the older person in a way that acknowledges their life and achievements, is the start of the relationship (Blood 2013: 16). Rekindling memories, whether through music, conversational topics, artefacts, photos, or arranged visits, is important both for the older user and for the social worker. Finding out and piecing together their narrative using triggers for recollection is as important for the social worker as it is for the person.

REFLECT AND DECIDE: CARE ELIGIBILITY CRITERIA

One result of service provision being driven by the rigid application of criteria is the situation in which John finds himself. He lives in a group home with three younger men, but when he reached 65 he was 'retired' from the day centre he had been attending for many years, while his case was transferred from the learning disability team to an older persons' team. The minibus still collects the other men each morning and the support staff at the group home say: 'He gets very angry and upset and we don't know how to explain it to him in a way that will make sense' (adapted from Ward 2012).

What reasons might justify the decision *not* to allow John to continue at the day centre? What reasons would justify his continuing there? Which is the more persuasive?

There is a difference, then, between independence and control. Independence is associated with a person remaining in (or returning to) their own home but does not mean doing everything for themselves. Control is more closely allied with having the choices and the capacity to make decisions over everyday issues that matter most. Having to decide from a field of many possibilities without a reliable guide to making decisions is stressful. Frail older people are more likely to have reduced capacity to make decisions as well as to execute those decisions independently (Rabiee 2013: 874). The importance of having someone on side to coordinate, navigate, advocate or advise is well established, but within a fragmented social care provision, hard to create. Blood *et al.* (2012) suggest a 'ringmaster' – a role which might be played by a relative, project manager or key worker – who coordinates the input of different services, filling gaps along the fault lines between them as necessary. Similarly Croucher and Bevan (2012) emphasise the importance of 'brokerage', or of staff making sure that individuals with higher support needs are able to take advantage of activities within housing with care schemes.

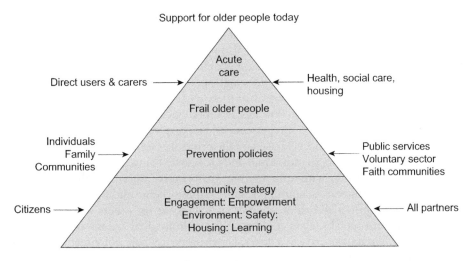

FIGURE 6.2   Inverting the triangle of care (author)

Socialisation and neighbourhood engagement

Engagement in social activities, social relationships and involvement in community are all recognised for maintaining and enhancing physical and mental health in older people (Hemingway and Jack 2013: 13). Next to concerns about health, the wish to engage in and be part of community affairs is a strong preference expressed across a number of surveys of older people. In disadvantaged districts of Manchester and Sheffield older residents expressed a strong attachment to their neighbourhood despite what was called 'locational disadvantage'. Surveys found that the higher the level of social contact, the higher the perceived quality of life and the lower the feelings of loneliness. Half those interviewed said they would choose to have more involvement if they could (ibid.).

On the other hand, demographic and social changes have weakened the capacity of support networks to provide emotional support such as social interaction, reassurance, cheering up and monitoring, as well as material support such as household jobs like preparing meals, cleaning, shopping for food, providing transport, bill paying and banking money. More women working, higher rates of divorce and greater geographical dispersion have made family networks more fragile (Keating *et al.* 2003). For those over 85 the loss of same-generation relatives and friends and the tendency to put energy into only the closest relationships (Keating *et al.* 2003) can undermine what a wider, more dispersed support network is capable of achieving.

A number of projects are underway which explore how communities need to adapt to an ageing society by keeping seniors engaged in neighbourhood life. Dementia Friendly communities, Strategy for Widowhood, Age UK's 'Village Agents' scheme, Brightlife in Cheshire – all build around the theme of supporting older people at a time of isolation and loneliness. The kinds of resources that are offered include lists of activities available in local community centres, information boards in town halls, adult education classes, care homes with space available for outside activities, and participatory research through which preferences and personal goals are articulated (Sinclair and Watson 2014). The local authority has a key role as service commissioner – especially social care budget holders – to support community interventions by revising rules to stimulate different models of provision and to ensure that smaller-scale, relationship-based services are not damaged. It should also be making sure that the range of services and benefits of different types of provision are clearly communicated – with front-line staff increasing take-up by spreading information, identifying carers who need support and pushing for continual development to meet local preferences. Gathering evidence on the effectiveness of various approaches and mixing core funding with other sources to ensure sustainability are two further council responsibilities (Bowers 2013).

These local options are loosely based on the principle of mutuality – people support-ing each other, contributing to individual and group wellbeing. But there are enormous challenges. One has to do with volunteering, the resource on which all these schemes rely. Recruiting volunteers, sustaining them, training them; finding 'core' volunteers who will shoulder principal responsibilities such as cover for others when they are off sick or take on liaison tasks when concern about an individual arises – is difficult work in its own right, but particularly in a general environment where volunteer levels overall are down because of time pressures on working adults.

Another challenge is even more difficult to resolve: will schemes based on mutuality sufficiently support carers? Care work, low-paid or unpaid as it is, can be exhausting, non-stop and filled with broken nights. When social care practice relies on informal carers from within the family, or on low-paid staff, women predominantly shoulder the main burden and responsibility for providing that care. As mentioned earlier, the argument made by feminists is that caring is essentially a gendered activity and that community care policies rely on this fact but do not acknowledge it. To refer only to 'carers', without also specifying the fact that the preponderance of caring is carried out by women, hides the exploitation on which the policy is based and without which it could not succeed.

REFLECT AND DECIDE: COHERENCE IN THE CARE SYSTEM FOR OLDER PEOPLE

Think Local, Act Personal – a national partnership spanning government and voluntary sec-tors – offers a map to navigate care support options. At the centre of the map is the personal 'cloud' of support to which older people will turn in the first instance – friends, family, GP, faith groups and support organisations with whom they are in contact. The cloud will pro-vide a range of services – from information to actual services – or so the TLAP maintains.

Do you think this is a realistic representation of the adult social care system? Does it gloss over aspects of reality? What is the difference between 'the cloud' and a social network? Why would the authors call it 'the cloud'?

CASE STUDY: BRIGHTLIFE

The Brightlife partnership is headed by Age UK Cheshire and spans a number of organisations and community groups, large and small, private, public and community-based. Its aim is to reduce social isolation among older people in the borough of Cheshire West and Chester and challenge assumptions about growing old by stimulating 'systemic change in services and behaviour through a strong brand'. At its core is a 'social pharmacy' through which, analogous to medical practice, social prescriptions to tackle isolation and build enduring social connections can be provided. These include local hubs to provide information, advice and access to services, increase accessibility to digital technology, increase volunteering and active citizenship among older people, and shape service markets around older people's actual needs, wants and aspirations. Sustainable models for befriending, peer mentoring and intergenerational activities are also among the objectives.

Older people are co-designing and co-producing Brightlife through design groups, the Older People's Alliance, Cheshire West Older People's network, community self-help groups and carers and relatives.

It is an ambitious project in line with the Better Care Fund, committed to testing and evaluating different ways of addressing social isolation. The challenges facing Brightlife are several: (i) the widespread social attitude that the first priority for old age is managing health and containing the cost of that; (ii) difficulties in recruiting, training and retaining a significant volunteer force on which the partnership will depend; (iii) the impact of continuing austerity on local authority expenditure, forcing smaller organisations to absorb costs within their personnel.

Dementia and social inclusion

Estimates suggest that, in England and Wales alone, there may be around 670,000 people currently living with dementia. Around 40 per cent of people aged 85 and over have a severe disability which makes it difficult for them to carry out various activities of daily living (Falkingham *et al.* 2010). There are difficulties applying the social model to dementia sufferers. Self-identity and agency, central to wellbeing, require self-reflection but that is often assumed to be lacking for those with dementia. Agency theory in particular has been criticised for concentrating on rationality, language, intention action and goal orientation (Hemmings and Kabesh 2013). The relative neglect of emotion, regarded as inferior to reason, has led to a divided view of self in which those cognitive abilities that remain are under-recognised while emotions are viewed as symptomatic of the illness. But emotion may be indicative of agency, especially within the institutionalised care regimes, low societal expectations and lack of opportunities to participate. The well-observed impact of music for example can lead to increased willingness to engage with care routines among those with even severe dementia (Boyle 2014: 1132).

CASE STUDY: LINDA

People with dementia often do not have the capacity to make key decisions completely on their own. On the other hand some can express their values or aspirations. Linda lacked the capacity to make financial decisions but she could identify the low priority she gave to wealth, in contrast to the emphasis she placed on her relationships. She would say 'You don't need a lot of money, as long as you have your happiness and one another and friends.'

Practice point: people with dementia should be given the opportunity to participate as fully as possible in decision-making processes relating to their present and future care. One way to do this is for the practitioner to explore preferences, values and aspirations in relation to the kinds of decisions that are to be made, even if the person is not able to make the actual decision themselves.

Important findings for practice emerge from the research on dementia and decision making. Too often choice, if offered at all, is restricted to low-level issues; available budgets are small and further hedged by constraints on what the money can be spent on. The low level of users' knowledge and their reluctance or inability to act, play an active role in their unwillingness to exit from care arrangements that they think are unsatisfactory (Boyle 2014). Too often users had not been able to choose their care provider agency to begin with. When they have choice they lack sufficient information on the care market to understand the relative merits of each option. Despite this there is satisfaction with the organisation from which they receive support. The gender of carers is important, as are religious and cultural preferences. Continuity of carers is also fundamental to a positive outcome. Users who establish close relationships with their care workers – and could request 'off-care plan' tasks – are especially appreciative (ibid.: 9). Austerity has bitten deep into the public consciousness; users know that public funding is limited and do not want carers to get into trouble for tasks they cannot carry out. The concept of 'time banking' is one means by which some flexibility in carers' schedules can be introduced.

KEY POINTS

❑   The adult social care system continues to evolve with an ever-increasing role for market-based provision. This leads to fragmentation and difficulty for social workers who want to pull together coherent, focused responses to tackling social exclusion. It also leads to the 'cartelisation' of providers – a few big private companies providing the bulk of care in given areas.

❑   Personalisation and individual budgets assist independence and control for those that can use them. They also reflect a consumerist approach to services and perhaps undermine collective solutions to adult social care needs.

❑   Those with disability and chronic ill health require advocacy and close support from practitioners when facing work capability assessments.

❑   Creating new or maintaining social networks is central to older people's wellbeing. The increase in loneliness and dementia among older people calls for community-based responses.

KEY READING

The social care environment is fast changing. For the time being, journal articles and reports are best placed to illuminate what is immediately going on.

Malcolm Carey's 'The fragmentation of social work and social care: some ramifications and a critique', *British Journal of Social Work*, Advanced Access, 29 September 2014, is a good place to start.
Imogen Blood's *A Better Life: Valuing Our Later Years* (Joseph Rowntree Foundation, 2013) lays out a broad, ecological understanding of growing old and the kinds of services required for the needs of older people.

There are insightful books that take a wider perspective:

Paul Bywaters, Eileen McLeod and Lindsey Napier have edited *Social Work and Global Health Inequalities: Practice and Policy Developments* (Policy Press, 2009), which clearly lays out the responsibilities of practitioners in tackling health inequality.
Michael Oliver, Bob Sapey and Pam Thomas have brought out the fourth edition of a classic, *Social Work with Disabled People* (Palgrave Macmillan, 2012).

CHAPTER 7

WORKING WITH DISADVANTAGED NEIGHBOURHOODS

THIS CHAPTER COVERS

- The process through which entire neighbourhoods become socially excluded.

- Approaches to building community strengths or 'capacity building' in support of residents and organisations determined to shape their own future.

- The importance of resident participation in any community development project and how to audit levels of participation.

- Strategies that help local services play a key role in reviving such areas, through partnerships and neighbourhood teams.

Social exclusion has a spatial or geographical dimension. In short, 'place' matters. This chapter explores the approaches and techniques of working with excluded neighbourhoods, helping to build structures and capacities on the ground enabling local residents to shape the renewal of their own localities.

WHY NEIGHBOURHOODS ARE IMPORTANT

As we saw in Chapter 1, the neighbourhood environment exerts an external influence over important dimensions of residents' lives such as child development, the feeling of security in old age, and the extent to which they want to participate in community affairs. As such 'the neighbourhood' has become a focus for a vast army of social scientists who are discussing at length both the various methods of gathering evidence on how neighbourhoods influence their residents and the specific ways by which that influence is exerted (Sampson 2013).

Neighbourhoods in decline

What cuts a neighbourhood off from the economic, social and political activity of the city or region within which it is located? Physical layout and the nature of the housing have something to do with it. The mass estates built for thousands of citizens after the Second World War were constructed around road layout and housing design that made looking after property difficult over the long term. From the mid-1960s, as the housing market was increasingly dominated by owner occupation, only those on relatively low income began to be concentrated on such estates. In the 1980s the collapse of industrial production in particular areas of the country – the northeast, the northwest, south Wales, for example – combined with the right of sitting tenants to buy council tenancies, accelerated the movement of those on low income to estates that were stigmatised locally.

Whether run by the local authority or, increasingly, by independent housing trusts or housing associations, social housing has today become an under-resourced, residual service for those individuals and families who cannot find accommodation in other parts of the housing system or do not have the resources to prevent their being assigned to the most stigmatised neighbourhoods. As a result, low-income households, which often need substantial supports, are channelled towards specific areas within a local authority. The consequence is polarisation within housing as the council estates provide for an increased proportion of deprived people and cater more exclusively for this group.

But poor housing is not the only factor in the social exclusion of neighbourhoods. As a result of the concentration of poor people living together, the social fabric of the estate – that is the way people relate to each other and the strength of local organisations such as churches or mosques – is also changed. In *Estates on the Edge*, Anne Power (1997) provides a good overview of how a range of negative pressures build up within large housing estates.

Figure 7.1 provides a model for the exclusionary process of a disadvantaged neighbourhood. It shows how a downward cycle develops as loss of jobs, services and commercial outlets combines with local conditions such as the layout and structure of an individual estate (for example with back-alley access to individual houses which facilitates burglary, and no onsite warden or manager) to produce a place with a poor reputation, and as families with high support needs and nowhere else to go take up shorter-term tenancies, creating transitory relationships and polarisation between young and old. These factors result in loss of confidence, abandoned property, loss of local activity, loss of authority and collapsing viability (Power 1997; Power and Mumford 1999: 81).

In working with deprived neighbourhoods, increasing the levels of participation by local residents – whether in local organisations and institutions, in decision making affecting the locality or in public services themselves – becomes an important goal. There are three reasons why. First, raising levels of participation ensures that the expressed needs of local residents are heard directly and are not shaped subtly by the interests of service providers or local officials. Second, local people can build skills

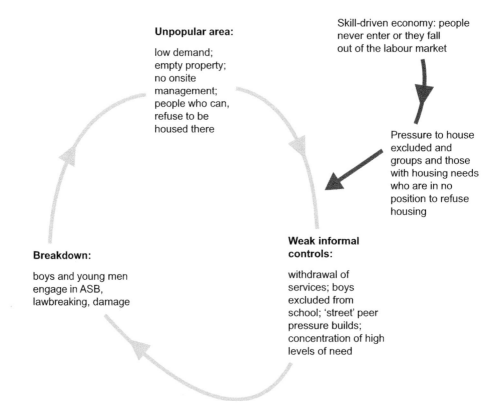

FIGURE 7.1   The cycle of exclusion (adapted from Power 1997)

and confidence that make them more effective in articulating their needs and demands and those of their neighbourhood. Third, as local residents learn to participate more effectively, their experience helps develop skills for further successful collaborations in solving local problems (Ferguson and Stoutland 1999: 51).

That is the theory at least. But there are practical barriers to participation by local residents, especially in low-income neighbourhoods, to take into consideration. Participation requires a great deal of time from people in time-poor environments; the alienating professional and managerial language that service providers often deploy is another factor, as is the burnout by those who regularly step forward to volunteer to sit on management boards or oversee yet another survey or attend yet another meeting – these are all obstacles to be surmounted by local people. A daunting range of skills are required to participate effectively: literacy and numeracy, negotiating skills to enable dialogue, confidence-building measures for groups new to participation, conflict and resolution skills to manage community organisations.

SOCIAL CAPITAL – A DEFINITION

'Social capital' is embodied in the social connections and networks of a given neighbourhood. It includes things like the level of activism in civic organisations, the degree of political involvement of residents and the vitality of local institutions such as churches or mosques. A number of indicators have been developed that show the extent of social capital in a given area. One such indicator is the proportion of individuals *not* involved in any civic organisation – whether political party, church, mosque or temple, trade union, tenants' association, club or social group. The lower that percentage, the lower the social capital of the neighbourhood. Other indicators include data on community safety such as the total number of burglaries (the lower the number, the more social capital), and the percentage of individuals expressing dissatisfaction with their neighbourhood (the higher the percentage, the less social capital there is) (Putnam 2001). Also included in an audit of social capital is the number of new community organisations associated with environmental or neighbourhood activism, social enterprises, credit unions and other participatory initiatives.

CAPACITY BUILDING

The common thread that runs through neighbourhood work is community building, now more frequently called 'capacity building'. Capacity building means helping a local area develop and strengthen local organisations, increasing levels of resident participation and engagement, and developing local leaders – all with the purpose of strengthening the neighbourhood to the point where it can take control of its own affairs and articulate issues important to it. When we refer to 'capacity' in relation to communities and neighbourhoods we mean their ability to act in particular ways, with specific faculties or powers to do or accomplish tasks (Chaskin *et al.* 2001). 'Capacity' enables local residents and organisations to engage in consultation, reach a consensus on important issues, articulate what the neighbourhood wants in meetings and in published reports. In general it means neighbourhoods can find 'voice' and 'agency' – to be heard, respected and have influence in decision-making forums that matter. If capacity building can be reduced to one phrase it would be 'learning to acquire and to use power and influence to secure certain democratically determined objectives'.

Concretely it includes training, personal skills development, mentoring and peer support for the ultimate benefit of the neighbourhood. Examples of capacity building initiatives include:

- Development of community vision and action plans.
- Negotiating a written service agreement with service providers.
- Ensuring community representatives chair and take up a majority of places on partnership boards and other forums of participation.
- Resident-led consultation including street meetings, door-to-door surveys and local planning events.
- Resourcing and supporting resident involvement in developing new local organisations to the point where residents themselves can manage the project and assets.

GETTING STARTED IN THE NEIGHBOURHOOD

There are several steps for practitioners to take to effectively engage with a specific neighbourhood. First, get to know the neighbourhood – its social and physical characteristics, its layout and hubs, the important institutions and associations, and the like. Second, think through clearly what the practitioner's role should be and that of the organisation she or he represents, and the relationship that is to be formed with prospective partners. Third, develop goals, objectives and plans in collaboration with a broad section of stakeholders in the neighbourhood.

Getting to know the neighbourhood: community profiling

It is essential to become familiar with the area. Talking to as many people and leaders of local organisations as you can provides the best way of building up a picture of who holds influence and what the effective networks are. This is often described as 'tacit' knowledge – the experiences and understanding of those who have lived in the locality for a long period of time or who have themselves large social networks along which knowledge – of events, people, institutions – is transmitted.

Gathering data

Certain elements of a neighbourhood's exclusion are easier to identify than others. Some, such as poor housing stock or level of unemployment, can be tracked quantitatively and show up in data provided by the local authority or the Office for National Statistics (ONS) – for example on the proportion of households where the head of household is not in work, the proportion of households that are overcrowded or the number of households living in temporary accommodation. There is also the hard data to collect and this task is now much easier than even ten years ago.

**CASE STUDY: CAPTURING RELEVANT
NEIGHBOURHOOD DATA**

Data on many aspects of community and neighbourhood life is now readily available from the Office for National Statistics. Go to www.statistics.gov.uk, click on 'Neighbourhood' and enter the name of the area, city, neighbourhood or specific streets you are interested in. The full range of data to do with socio-economic status of the area becomes available. Data that previously would have taken months to accumulate is now only a couple of mouse clicks away. Search for data on the neighbourhood or area where you are regularly involved and see whether it confirms your own estimates as to: (i) how many adults have a work-limiting disability; (ii) how many people are living on benefits; and (iii) the type and number of crimes committed.

Local data, focused on only a few streets, is also available. These so-called 'super output areas' (SOAs) bring together a high volume of information provided for small target areas. It may be possible to define your neighbourhood or district precisely by adding together several output areas. SOA data provides multiple data sets on key areas of neighbourhood life, which includes numbers of households with limiting long-term illness and dependent children, number of lone-parent households with dependent children, breakdown of ethnicity, economic activity and gender. To access this information from the Office for National Statistics website, practitioners need only a postcode or the name of an area they wish to explore.

MAPPING A NEIGHBOURHOOD

Neighbourhoods are dynamic, contested places 'created by the particular interaction of flows and processes such as social relationships, economics and politics operating at varying levels from the local to the global' (Holland et al. 2011: 691). Individuals and families are enmeshed, as ecological theory tells us, within these neighbourhood forces.

Since the 2008 recession, inequality has intensified – in levels of wealth but also in housing where wealth has transferred from the poorest to the comfortably well-off in dramatic fashion. We are also just beginning to see all the possible connections between housing, society, inequality and health (Dorling 2013). Using a large-scale map or Google Earth, plot housing tenures – council, social housing, owner-occupied and privately rented. Identify recent transfers from public housing authorities to private landlords and owner-occupation. Using the map, reflect on the housing needs for those under 25 years of age and for those over 75 years of age and whether or not, given the current housing, those needs can be met.

Accumulating vital accurate information is useful in subsequent negotiations with other stakeholders, for project proposals and funding applications. It is surprising how fast you can build up your familiarity with the networks in the neighbourhood. Soon you should be able to put together, for example, a rough neighbourhood network map and a list of local organisations with the names of individuals prominent within them.

Thinking through the practitioner's role

Before beginning any concerted neighbourhood work it is important to resist the temptation to undertake some form of immediate engagement and instead to think through what the objectives are of the work ahead. That temptation to begin immediately – by making all kinds of contacts and carving a path of your own strewn with suggestions for residents to chew over – is especially strong for those new to neighbourhood activity.

It is unlikely that as part of a larger effort to tackle social exclusion on an estate a community practitioner would be given an open-ended brief to do 'community social work' without broad objectives already in place. Such initiatives are always complex projects and often tied to larger partnerships. These extend over long periods of time, so you, your team and your agency will want to discuss what its contribution as part of a long-term strategy will be and how it will be able to sustain the effort. You will need to think through in advance what is possible within your existing roles and responsibilities and also how those roles and responsibilities might be altered to incorporate explicitly some form of neighbourhood involvement. Are you and your agency really willing to work in partnership and perhaps to let others receive credit for a well-handled project? Will your agency provide funding to local residents' groups even though it means diverting funding from elsewhere? Are you able to merge activities with other service agencies who may be identified as a 'lead body'? How far do you think resident participation and control should go? Are you willing to set aside notions of professional expertise and control to allow residents and their organisations to develop their own projects and approaches although they may diverge from your notion of what ought to happen?

For any particular project a broad brief may already have been formulated by your agency, or by a local partnership board. But the basis of your entry into the neighbourhood still requires explanation and negotiation. You will need to know where you fit within the broad outlines of a given project or emerging regeneration plan. Explaining what you see as your role and how it fits with the aspirations of local people will be a distinct challenge. The local priest, Bangladeshi youth leader, activist nun, tough-minded pensioner who heads the local tenants' association, local councillor, manager of the local women's centre, committee raising funds for a mosque – will all have influence and will all want to know what you are about.

REFLECT AND DECIDE: HOW FAR ARE COMMUNITIES INVOLVED?

Burns *et al.* (2004) have developed their own ratings scale on which to chart how much influence communities have over particular neighbourhood projects: 9 = lip service – participation amounts to nothing; 8 = consultation around pre-arranged options; 7 = provision of high-quality information; 6 = genuine consultation; 5 = community has formal advisory role; 4 = limited delegation of control over decision making; 3 = substantial delegation of control to community; 2 = community control over all activities within agreed conditions; 1 = community ownership of all assets.

Think of a major 'partnership' project in which community participation is emphasised. Using the scale above, note the extent of participation in each of the following functions:

- Policy making.
- Strategic planning including budget decisions.
- Commissioning – who gets funded.
- Budgetary control – who has day-to-day responsibility as well as overall accountability.
- Managing staff – including appointment, appraisal and training.
- Identifying objectives and performance indicators.
- Planning individual projects.
- Managing individual projects.

(adapted from Burns *et al.* 2004)

Developing goals, extending participation

The capacity to draw out and utilise the knowledge, motivation and viewpoints of local citizens is a prerequisite for a community's feeling of ownership and having a stake in neighbourhood-based services.

Finding community representatives

Strong levels of participation provide the foundation for public support of public and voluntary services. It comes through many different channels, such as local councillors, user groups, or residents' associations, or through links with local institutions such as schools, GP surgeries, ante-natal classes, sheltered accommodation and libraries. The public may voice opinion at meetings, through questionnaires and surveys on paper or online, or letters to the editor of the local paper. Shaping services has many decision points and should provide many entry points for local citizens to participate. There is no set formula for achieving good enough participation, but the public soon detects when it is mechanistic or done out of duty or as a result of requirement. The challenge for services in Xavier de Sousa Briggs's fine phrase is to find 'the will and the way' to forms of participation that mean something to local people (Briggs 2002).

Mohan and Bulloch argue that actual non-engagement is quite limited – few people contribute nothing at all – but their research also indicates that a 'civic core', a relatively small group in a locality, contribute a large proportion of formal civic engagement (Mohan and Bullock 2012). They looked at three dimensions of civic participation – volunteering, charitable donation and participation in community groups. They then analysed citizenship data of nearly 30,000 people – how many hours they spent giving unpaid help in a month, how much money they gave to charity in a month, and how many types of civic association they took part in over the previous twelve months. Informal volunteering, for example helping neighbours, was not captured by the study. They found that just over a third of the population provided 90 per cent of the volunteering hours, 80 per cent of the amount given to charity and 90 per cent of participation in organisations. Looking further into the data they discovered that 9 per cent of the population contributed half of volunteer hours.

REFLECT AND DECIDE: MAPPING LOCAL BARRIERS TO PARTICIPATION

A thorough audit of participation in any initiative or project will not only reveal a great deal about the project with which you are involved but will also tell you a lot about how to maximise participation in other projects. Burns and colleagues have put together a handbook for assessing the degree and effectiveness of participation that is applicable to virtually all projects. There are several main tools for carrying out an audit of participation:

- Baseline exercises mapping the extent of participation at a given point in time.
- Checklists of activities and approaches that contribute to effective community involvement.
- Questions that need to be asked if community involvement is to be effective.
- Scales to help practitioners and stakeholders to think through the quality and extent of the participation activities they are planning in the future.
- A 'decision trail' to track whether particular matters raised by local residents got into the decision-making arena, how these matters were decided upon and by whom, and finally whether or not they were actually implemented.

(Burns *et al.* 2004)

There are several implications of the existence of a civic core that social care practitioners involved in community groups – or who are hoping to outsource their services – should bear in mind. First, there clearly exists in many communities a relatively small group of people whose energy can be drawn on – willing to take on an outsized burden of responsibility in forming independent, community-based services. They have the skills, they have the time, and they have the motivation and interest to do so. Second, this core can become self-perpetuating, or at least appear as the 'same old faces' to others who may be thinking of taking on some of the tasks associated with a particular project. Third, there is the risk of burnout in these key civic participants; those constituting the civic core are not indestructible – they are often in their early sixties and recently retired but may be subject to health difficulties or loss of energy. There are also problems of succession – how projects are handed on to others. The two are not unrelated – as those who want to step down may feel unable to do so because there is no one else to take up the set of responsibilities. For those in the public sector these factors suggest that back-up and support will help the civic core carry its responsibilities.

Facilitation

Facilitation differs from mediation because, unlike the latter, which tries to solve disabling conflicts with community groups, it aims to explore complexity, and achieve better thinking and clearer positions on matters considered important by local citizens. Facilitation is a set of skills that focus on getting an effective process in place for participatory group decision making. It seeks to overcome the flaws that dominate group decision making which stifle creative decision making and create conflict. Flaws typically encountered in local area groups include:

- Value judgements inhibit spontaneity and deter others from expressing their views on matters significant to them.
- Exploration of complexity is discouraged.
- Emphatically expressed views hold greater sway in a public discussion than tentative or awkwardly put views.
- Rushed action plans and tight deadlines answer the need to be seen to do something.
- Considered, deliberative thinking is ignored as counter-productive.

(Kaner *et al.* 1996)

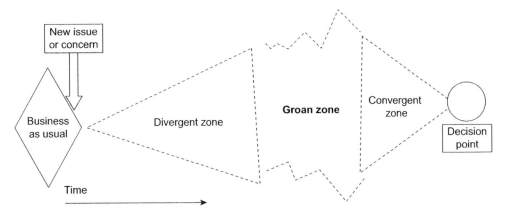

FIGURE 7.2   The 'groan zone' (Kaner *et al.* 1996; reproduced with permission from New
Society Publishers)

Participatory groups respond to these problems. Opposing viewpoints are given time and space and are allowed to coexist; people are supportive and draw each other out ('is this what you mean?'); people listen to the ideas of others because they know their own ideas will be heard; members of the group can accurately represent each other's points of view – even if they disagree with them; when the group reaches a decision it reflects a wide range of perspectives. The facilitator encourages everyone to do their best thinking (Kaner *et al.* 1996). Inevitably new issues, differing personalities, beliefs and opinions affect the proceedings with a rising sense of frustration and the feeling that the process is going nowhere. This is the 'groan zone' phase – which a good facilitator will help the group (committee, task force) to overcome.

USING VOLUNTEERS

Services have to increasingly rely on volunteers. This is partly positive – services that are more innovative and community-based draw on the efforts of local people in a non-paid capacity. It is also partly negative – the local authority has simply had to withdraw from the field and local, voluntary efforts have had to fill the void. Volunteers shoulder weighty, complex responsibilities in many different ways – peer support for parents, youth work, in day centres for older people, early years care and education, school pupils mentoring their peers, in credit unions, befriending schemes for the lonely and isolated, dementia care schemes. Volunteers also give enormous amounts of time and energy taking part in executive boards of neighbourhood initiatives and community forums of all descriptions. Some national organisations build their entire service around what their volunteers, all of whom have been trained to a uniform high level, have to offer: Home Start provides parent mentoring; Citizens Advice Bureaux provide advice on benefits, Age UK on services for older people.

Volunteering has its rewards – social involvement, helping others, giving a structure to life for adults in periods of transition, acquisition of new skills. Adults as volunteers can play an acknowledged role in the community while young people gain valuable experience and perhaps a qualification. But as society has profoundly changed in the last twenty years there are also steep barriers to volunteering. Time pressures inhibit parents who are working and raising a family. Grandparents are called on to perform caring roles within their own families and no longer have the time for volunteering in the community.

Perhaps more important than time is the feeling of being exploited or having to commit to great responsibilities. Local authorities have cut back their services to such an extent that front-line roles in youth clubs, day centres, visiting schemes, local shops, libraries and hospitals fall heavily on volunteers. Councils contract out their services to other entities which in turn are cheaper to run because they rely on volunteers (Rabin and McKenzie 2014). Compulsory volunteering, as required for job seekers under Universal Credit, also undermines the sense of goodwill behind volunteering. Another source of feeling exploited is that core volunteering falls on the relatively few to provide services for the many. Thus an informal 'free-rider' problem is set up – people who are content to use a service that volunteers provide but do not contribute by volunteering themselves. Finally, perhaps there is a change in mood in society as a whole as individualisation makes further inroads – individual actions are more closely judged on the immediate rewards they bring, and altruistic behaviour –'doing good' – does not yield that kind of reward.

REFLECT AND DECIDE: RECRUITING VOLUNTEERS

A youth centre in a small rural town runs a two-hour session every Friday night during school terms. As many as fifty kids attend between the ages of 9 and 13. The centre has been running on an all-volunteer basis for twelve years. Core volunteers, the regulars who turn up each and every week, are small in number and getting older. Members of the core are committed to staying in place during school terms, forgoing travel or visits to their own grown offspring. This core is supplemented by half a dozen young people from school years 10 and 11 who come regularly to help.

Efforts, however, to recruit from parents of those who attend have proved disappointing – the great majority are unwilling to commit to even one evening a term. Why is this so? What do you think the parents who refuse to volunteer say to themselves to convince themselves that it is OK *not* to volunteer *at all*? How might more volunteers be recruited?

Most volunteer recruitment strategies aim at one of two demographics: young people and those in their sixties nearing or in retirement. Parents of children and young people are largely regarded as out of reach. Volunteering is heavily gendered – men provide only 20 per cent of all volunteers. To encourage recruitment the Local Government Association has suggested enticements such as a 10 per cent council tax reduction; others have suggested free child care or small payments as 'expenses'.

But volunteering is not without its costs or limitations to the organisation that uses it. Recruiting, training and managing an unpaid workforce costs money and time. As roundtables and surveys have shown, volunteers are attracted and motivated by a range of factors and, as demographics shift, these are likely to become more complex.

The voluntary sector will need to become more adept at handling them. The goodwill that the voluntary sector taps into when it engages its band of volunteers can dry up quickly due to societal shifts, feelings of exploitation, the politicisation of volunteering and changing perceptions of volunteering.

The more dependent a charity is on volunteer time, the more they will need to focus on how, in an ageing society, the 'life-course' changes for their volunteers. People will expect to see charities adapt to their changing needs and capacity, and respond to the skills and energy that they bring. Even small gestures, for example inviting volunteers to staff away days, are a step in the right direction (Rabin and McKenzie 2014).

Social work as a professionalised activity has only relatively recently embraced the positive role that volunteers play, both in the peer-level expertise they have to offer and the role they play in providing social 'glue' in the locality. The first wave of radical social work in the 1970s was suspicious of volunteers as a force for undermining wages and potential threat to trade union solidarity. On the other hand community social work as envisioned in the 1980s began explicitly to acknowledge the role for volunteers. In the twenty-first century it is clear that the ensemble of social care activities could not be carried out without volunteers, with local charities and community organisations, befriending and visiting schemes, youth work and day centres all depending on them.

An emphasis on neighbourhood work means that use of volunteers should become more systematic:

- Volunteering provides individuals with a means of expressing values that are important to them. Recruitment to support a specific cause or service within the programme might have greater appeal. It is probably a mistake to couch the encouragement of volunteering only in the context of 'work-readiness' or tackling 'workless households', although it may have that longer-term effect for individuals.
- Recruitment and retention of volunteers go together. Poor recruitment practices lead to increased turnover. To aid recruitment, meaningful job assignments could be prepared – with some specification of skill level. There should be some matching of would-be volunteers to specific skills that need to be developed for those particular roles.
- Many first-time volunteers have lofty expectations of what the experience will be like – and so some work around managing those expectations is worthwhile. Volunteers placed in inappropriate jobs will be dissatisfied and quit. Volunteers recruited ineffectively may then form the wrong impression of the organisation and spread this by word of mouth.
- Widen the number of projects that rely on volunteer workers and provide them with the responsibility to seek out and recruit volunteers. Everyone in the programme should see recruitment as part of their duties. Facilitate the connections between those already serving as volunteers and those who might do so. Current volunteers may provide friends or contacts that they can recruit and then offer emotional and task-oriented support.
- Most people become volunteers after being asked to volunteer by a friend, family member or a person known to them who is already volunteering. People are flattered when asked to volunteer, even if they decline, although research tells us that 90 per cent of people who are directly invited to volunteer agree to do so.
- Finding and using male volunteers is one key way of introducing men into the lives of children. Set up recruitment campaigns around what that volunteering

activity could mean for the men who take it up: for instance that they will gain valuable experience working with children, for their own parenting skills or as an area of future employment. High schools, colleges and universities are possible sources for male volunteers. Service environments can be confusing to the newcomer, so some direction as to the specific type of activity the male volunteer could take on – whether in the reading corner or on the playground – would help orient the newly recruited male volunteer.

(adapted from Wymer and Starnes 2001 and Ewing *et al*. 2002)

COMMUNITY ORGANISING

Community organising gets to the heart of the problem that faces all community-level activities: who holds power and how the relatively powerless can attain power within an environment that systematically denies it to them. As one organiser has summed it up: 'It is because individuals in isolation have little power that a power analysis focuses mainly on institutions and on the people who play consequential roles in them' (Stout 2010: 55).

The school of community organising founded by Saul Alinsky (1909–1972) and active today through vibrant organisations such as the Citizen Organising Foundation in the UK and the Industrial Areas Foundation in the US, begins any organising initiative with an analysis of the distribution of power in a community. A power analysis determines what resources, institutional and otherwise, ordinary people have at their disposal when exercising their right to engage in the democratic process, resources that are apart from economic and governmental institutions. The aim of a citizen's organisation is to create a force, independent of government and corporate power, sufficient to influence vital decisions in the arenas where those decision are made. In so far as the disadvantaged are politically isolated from one another, they tend to be unaware of the benefits that organised political power can bring to them (Stout 2010: 58).

SAUL ALINSKY'S RULES FOR RADICAL COMMUNITY ORGANISERS

Here are seven of Saul Alinsky's thirteen rules for radicals. They take advantage of the patterns of weakness, arrogance, repeated mistakes, and miscalculations that large dominant organisations, whether corporate or public, and their leaderships make:

- Power is not only what you have but what the target thinks you have.
- Never go outside the expertise of your people. Feeling secure stiffens the backbone.
- Whenever possible, go outside the expertise of the target. Look for ways to increase their insecurity, anxiety, and uncertainty.
- Make the target live up to its own book of rules. If the rule is that every letter [or email] gets a reply, send thousands.

- Ridicule, especially against organisational leaders, is a potent weapon. There's no defence. It's irrational. It's infuriating. It also works as a key pressure point to force concessions.
- A good tactic is one your people enjoy. They'll keep doing it without urging and come back to do more. They'll even suggest better ones.
- Keep the pressure on. Never let up. Keep trying new tactics to keep the opposition off balance. As the target masters one approach, hit them with something new.

(adapted from Alinsky 1971)

The bedrock of organising is the one-to-one meeting, the aim of which is to build a relationship, a concept that is familiar to social workers. However, instead of an essentially private relationship convened as an interview to discuss matters in confidence with the user, the relational meeting is an encounter between individuals that is face to face *for the purpose of exploring the development of a public relationship*. The organiser is 'searching for talent, energy, insight and relationships; where these are present you have found some power to add to your public collective' (Chambers 2003: 45). Without these meetings people cannot forge lasting public relationships based on solid social knowledge or build lasting citizen's organisations. The relational meeting brings up stories that reveal people's deepest commitments and the experiences that give rise to them. The aim is to then fuse these many relationships to create a durable, diverse alliance of people and the institutions of which they are members, such as mosques, churches or trade unions, and community associations, to the point where, collectively, they have the influence, skills and resources to articulate demands and apply pressure on those who can meet those demands.

The relational meeting draws directly on bedrock social work skills – the ability to form relationships through use of self, critical listening, and probing for what a person values and what motivates them. The difference is wholly to do with the purpose the relationship is put to. With a user the relationship endeavours to solve the problems and difficulties facing that user, drawing on their strengths and providing support as needed. The impact essentially is personal to the user and their family. In community organising the aim is public accomplishment – finding commonalities and shared views on issues and problems facing residents across a community or neighbourhood, and welding those into an organisation that can articulate its demands and press those demands in the public arena.

CASE STUDY: CITIZENS UK

Citizens UK is a network of broad-base organisations that runs its own training programme for local activists and leaders. In a week-long series of seminars, discussions and role plays, trainees are exposed to the practicalities of mounting a local 'action': from one-to-one meetings in order to find common ground to highlighting local issues and holding to account those with the power to tackle those issues. The training coincides with a chance to watch community action in progress: for instance an accountability session when citizens call on their local officials or councillors to agree to particular actions. This provides an opportunity to assess the application of the principles and techniques they have learned in the workshop. But the purpose of the training is also to teach the wider obligations and responsibilities of civic action. Their curriculum includes several key learning points:

- Knowing how to clarify the difference between public and private roles for an individual, and how to conduct yourself and meet your responsibilities with regard to the former, not mixing or confusing the two.
- Learning to respond to public officials by developing the skills needed to hold your ground in a meeting or negotiating session.
- The nature of power – that power is both unilateral (that is, directive, compelling and coercive) and relational (built up through association, building consensus and finding common interests and motivations among diverse groups of individuals and organisations).
- Skills for successful 'relational organising' which is built on listening and engagement with residents in small formats such as one-to-one sessions or small house meetings.
- Applying pressure: how to build countervailing power locally to help in bargaining with city officials and politicians.
- The nature and conduct of negotiation – learning to balance conciliation with the application of pressure.

(adapted from Citizens UK 2015; Chambers 2004)

The Brazilian educationist, Paolo Freire (b. 1927, d. 1997), continues to have an outsized influence on the way community development is an educative process. He argued that perceptions of powerlessness erode hope and create a 'culture of silence' that goes some way to explaining why the poor seem to accept the harshness of their lives and settle for explanations of individual failure rather than collective oppression.

Freire believed that every human being is capable of critically engaging their world once they begin to question the contradictions that shape their lives through a process of what he called 'conscientisation' – the process of becoming aware of contradictions whether political, cultural, socio-economic. The worker seeks to draw out from people's experiences what the most pressing problems are and to 'problematise' them, i.e. look at the complexity and their relationship to forces well beyond the power of the individual to change on their own. Freire promoted a 'critical pedagogy' through which every process of community organising has to contain a process of education. Education cannot be neutral: either it serves the *reproduction* of the dominant order or creates space for *production* in which citizens learn to think for themselves. Such a pedagogy should include the basic skill of dialogue – a mutual and reciprocal form of communication, embodying respect and relationship. Otherwise community development work would only begin to recreate another, albeit different system which would impose its own values, assumptions, perceptions.

Mendes (2009) sees much in common between social work and community development and provides a concise exposition of the relationship between them, including an account of how social work constructs community development and vice versa. Interestingly, he relates the hostility of some community development educators and practitioners towards social work to a false construction of community development as inherently radical and social work as inherently conservative. In reality, both have conservative and radical components [and] many contemporary programmes such as neighbourhood renewal are based on working within our existing socio-political system rather than developing strategies to explicitly challenge social structures.

(Mendes 2009: 249)

COMMUNITY-LEVEL SERVICES AND COMMUNITY-BASED SERVICES

When looking at the wide range of approaches and interventions for work with neighbourhoods it is helpful to distinguish between those interventions that are community-based and those that are at community level (Barnes *et al.* 2006). Both provide services to people and both are geographically based but they work in different ways and with different objectives.

Community-level interventions aim to improve levels of wellbeing across a given locality or neighbourhood as their main objective and in the course of doing so may well assist individuals or families. This type of intervention, Barnes and her colleagues argue, is based on the conviction 'that social problems, especially those created by disadvantage, are best dealt with by "capacity building" [in] the community rather than by identifying individuals with problems and providing services to them' (Barnes *et al.* 2006: 87). The assumption behind community-level interventions is that a vigorous community with the capacity to solve its own problems will improve wellbeing for all who live there. Community-level action assists the community in acquiring certain assets – strengthening community groups, strengthening social networks, providing a new service open to all, gaining voice and sense of agency and effectiveness.

Community-based interventions, by contrast, aim to meet the needs of individuals and families through services and supports delivered in the community. Such local services are typically available through common access points, such as local schools, health clinics or local offices, or through drop-in centres and outreach work. Referrals tend to be self-initiated and informally dealt with. The aim is to meet specified needs, offer support for specified difficulties or provide information. Sexual health clinics, carers support groups, and psychological services for young people are all examples. The outcome of this kind of intervention is change in levels of wellbeing for individuals and families, while any capacity building for the community as a whole is a by-product of the service.

Some service providers do both because they aim to increase community capacity and at the same time offer services and support to individuals and families. Indeed there is a close connection between the two (Barnes *et al.* 2006). Sure Start children's centres, when they were well funded and widely available, provide a good example. Their objective was – and for those that remain still is – to raise standards of parenting and child development across the whole of the neighbourhood in which they are situated. They also provide services to individual families – child care, speech therapy, support for mothers with post-natal depression. Dementia-friendly activities also do both – educating their communities on responding to those with dementia while offering a home visiting service for those afflicted. In practice, then, it is often difficult to pinpoint where the community-based service ends and the community-level intervention begins.

Social work has had perennial difficulties in engaging in community-level interventions. This is in part because of its belief in the efficacy of individually oriented casework but also because of pressure to respond to safeguarding crises and the rationalisation of new public management from the 1990s which separated political from individual actions. As a result, social work education has shown less interest in community social work (Dixon and Hoatson 1999). This has produced a paradox whereby social work committed itself to combating oppression in its value base at the same time as dispensing with the one important element needed to bring that work into focus: skills for community and neighbourhood engagement. However the occupational spaces of social work are changing, in part because of legal mandates across a whole range of services to involve communities – participation, empowerment of local people. As these mandates are constrained by austerity there also needs to be a long-term strategic commitment to tackle the visible effects of the restructuring of the welfare state and open up the professional agenda to include grappling with the 'deep-seated socio-economic conditions that characterize the lives' of users (Das *et al.* 2015: 3). Social workers can and should be important allies within community development work, argue Das and colleagues, particularly in partnership with community organisations. In Northern Ireland individualised services are simply inadequate to undertake the anti-sectarian work needed among disempowered communities; only through community development can power inequalities in structure and institutions be examined, hidden assumptions uncovered and marginal voices emerge (ibid.: 11).

THE JAY REPORT ON CHILD SEXUAL EXPLOITATION IN ROTHERHAM

Alexis Jay pointed to the difference between the 'social work model' – social workers holding individual caseloads and pressured by statutory functions – adopted by the council and the 'community development model' of Risky Business, the voluntary organisation that had tried to publicise the problem of child sexual exploitation. The latter, she argued, was more suitable for tackling the scale of CSE in Rotherham.

(Jay 2014)

KEY POINTS

❑   Neighbourhoods are important; disadvantaged neighbourhoods have specific effects on the lives of residents.

❑   Disadvantaged neighbourhoods can be excluded in their entirety – alienated from the larger geographical community of which they should be a part. Much of a social worker's practice will be based in neighbourhoods such as these.

❑ Social work has generally privileged the importance of its work with individuals and families but as awareness of 'neighbourhood effects' expands so does the need to focus on community interventions.

❑ Getting to know the neighbourhood – mapping, profiling, gathering social data – is an essential first step to increasing resident participation in projects and service policy direction.

❑ Broad-base community organising techniques focus explicitly on power – who holds it and how to acquire it.

❑ There is a difference between community-level and community-based projects. Both acknowledge the importance of neighbourhoods and respond to their strengths and weaknesses.

KEY READING

Margaret Ledwith, *Community Development in Action: Putting Freire into Practice* (Policy Press, 2015). Ledwith links community development to the powerful educative role that Freire developed.

Jeffrey Stout, *Blessed Are the Organised: Grassroots Democracy in America* (Princeton University Press, 2010). Stout is in the mould of Saul Alinsky. Alinsky's *Rules for Radicals* is still worth reading. Both books relate to the US.

John Pierson, *Going Local: Working in Communities and Neighbourhoods* (Routledge, 2007) develops community practice for social workers across a number of domains.

CHAPTER 8

SOCIAL WORK AND SOCIAL EXCLUSION IN RURAL AREAS

THIS CHAPTER COVERS

- Definition of what is 'rural' and how that contrasts with 'urban'.

- Types of social exclusion particular to villages and small towns.

- The constraints on organising service systems for dispersed populations in rural areas.

- Service approaches that overcome barriers to inclusion in rural areas.

In the early 1900s Britain became an urban nation when, for the first time for any country, more people lived in cities than in the countryside. This was the long-term result of the population shift arising from the industrial revolution that had begun in the late eighteenth century. (Population experts estimate that, globally, a majority of the world's population for the first time lived in cities rather than rural areas in 2007.) The move to the city of course had profound consequences for the countryside; indeed the changes unleashed continue to impact rural life. This chapter discusses these changes in recent years and the distinctively rural forms of exclusion created in their wake.

Many of the approaches to tackling exclusion in the countryside are the same as outlined in earlier chapters – the focus on poverty, social network functioning, user participation and neighbourhood-based services. The aim of this chapter is to alert readers to the constraints that beset the delivery of rural services – time, distance, and dispersed populations – and look at ways that these can be overcome.

Historically, the countryside had been a place of extreme physical exclusion – expulsion, incarceration, loss of rights. Enclosures of common land in England and clearances of crofters in the Scottish highlands, together with strict anti-poaching laws,* deprived local populations of resources for raising livestock and grain that once were open to all. Famine combined with rapid industrialisation and the effects of the new Poor Law in the nineteenth century caused widespread forced migration from all parts of the British Isles but particularly from Ireland.

This was exclusion on an epic scale and took place against a backdrop of peasants dependent on common land for survival and indentured farm labourers living in tied cottages while working for chronically low wages. They made a subsistence living only by working their small personal plots of land. Once these were taken away they were often reduced to absolute poverty. Attempts by farm labourers to protest against the rise in the price of bread, a key staple for energy, or to forestall wage cuts through unionisation, were repressed throughout much of the nineteenth century. The local magistracy representing the established church and landed interests rigorously upheld strict social and legal codes based on the hierarchy of the established order. Anyone who opposed this order was deemed alien to morality and undermining propriety and possession of property. The histories, then, of many rural areas are a story of poverty, exploitation and dependence on the locally powerful.

Moreover, class division, social stratification and inequality remain, as recent studies of gentrification of rural areas have shown. Class analysis still illuminates the processes of social change in the countryside – the relevance of class as an expression of exploitation combines with issues of recognition, identity and cultural difference, albeit with no expectation that a 'class consciousness' emerges from this, not at least among the exploited and excluded (Shucksmith 2012; Phillips 2011).

URBAN AND RURAL CONTRASTS

Contrasts between rural and urban life remained a source of investigation and social thought even as the number of people living in the countryside declined. Given the extent of the social problems that emerged from cities – whether poor sanitation, overcrowded and poorly built housing, or unemployment and mass poverty – commentary contrasting urban problems with the timeless nature of rural life became a dominant theme. Ferdinand Tönnies, a German sociologist, over a hundred years ago captured some of these differences in terms that were influential in British and American social science and have proved remarkably durable. He argued that in a rural 'community' (gemeinschaft) social order is based on multiple social ties. People know each other across different roles – as parents, neighbours, employees, friends or kin. In contrast, urban residents live in 'association' (gesellchaft) and know each other only in single, specialised roles either as neighbours or employees, but not both. Social relations within gesellschaft, Tönnies thought, are more calculating and contractual (Tönnies 2001).

Such thinking about rural communities remains influential and some generalisations built on it still abound. The countryside is said to be a place of face-to-face communities where the boundary between private and public life is blurred and where individuals live under close scrutiny by others. 'Village hall' politics is dominated by

---

*In the eighteenth century the so-called 'Black Act' made many petty crimes against property a hanging offence and Britain had for a time the greatest number of capital crimes in Europe (Thompson 1977).

'in-groups' that have been in place for years and underpinned by a social structure shaped in an era of landed and agricultural interests where hunting and field sports were prominent and notions of economic growth powerfully influenced by farming practices. Recent stereotypes have also emerged – for example the countryside as lacking diversity in its ethnic and cultural make-up, or its public services as lagging behind in innovation and outlook.

Changing nature of the countryside

The social profile of the countryside has changed, however, undermining many of the old stereotypes. The boom in productivity in agriculture brought with it a decline in the number of agricultural workers required for agricultural production – employment in agriculture has declined by some 30 per cent since the mid-1980s – and at the same time has brought about greater diversity in land use. The trend of the population at large that views the countryside either as a place for recreation or residence from which to commute to work, has introduced new elements into a social mix that had been long dominated by farming.

Alongside this the availability of land and premises for industrial parks and small businesses has further diversified the rural economy. Rural employees are now more likely to find work in manufacturing (25 per cent), tourism (9 per cent) or retailing (7 per cent), than in agriculture (6 per cent) (DEFRA 2003). Around 73 per cent of jobs in rural Britain are now in services, compared with 60 per cent in 1981. Rural areas have thus shared in the general shift to a service-based economy in which the information and knowledge-based industries play an increasing role (Shucksmith 2000).

Migration *into* rural areas is now significant with some 60,000 people migrating per year between 1991 and 2002. But this masks other dramatic changes in rural demographics. The rural population is ageing with the number of people aged 65 or over increasing by some 12 per cent (161,000) in the same ten-year period, while the number of people aged 16–29 decreased by 237,000 or 18 per cent. The rates of net loss of 16–19- and 20–24-year-olds are especially high for smaller villages and hamlets. In Scotland rural out-migration is predominantly an exodus of young people (Jamieson and Groves 2008). Although difficult to quantify precisely, a significant proportion of migrant workers from Eastern European countries have arrived in rural areas, with, for example, a need to provide English as a second language for school pupils. Concerns, however, have been raised about the supposed strain placed on public services through catering for an expanded population. This is seen as particularly problematic in rural areas. From a social and cultural perspective, migrants might be seen as unwelcome neighbours 'out of place', leading separate lives and unsettling senses of local and national identity. Seen differently it can be argued that Eastern European migrants have precipitated a degree of cultural exchange and enriched the fabric of those areas in which they have settled (Storey 2013).

The phenomenon clearly highlights the tensions between a global labour market and ideas of the local. It is also the case that these more recent migrants display high levels of mobility, with evidence of considerable movement back and forth between home and host countries. Aided by modern communication systems migrants are retaining close connections (both real and virtual) to 'home'. There appear to be high levels of what has been termed 'population churn' with indications of high levels of return migration as well as internal movement by international migrants within the UK (Dennett and Stillwell 2008).

In England the recession of 2008 was a catalyst for tens of thousands who moved to the countryside in its wake. Better broadband connections meant that many could relocate and continue working remotely as they looked for different job opportunities and lifestyles. DEFRA reported that over a hundred thousand people moved to the countryside in 2010–2011 (DEFRA 2012). All together it calculated that some 12.7 million people, a quarter of England's population, were living in rural areas: 50 per cent were aged 45 or more (compared to 36 per cent in cities).

As a consequence of these movements, the rural economy is diversifying, with some of the hallmarks of growing affluence, but losing its youth. On the whole unemployment tends to be lower, car ownership higher, and housing conditions better than in urban areas. Rural-based industrial estates draw their employees not from the locality but from towns and more distant commuter belts.

Changes in the rural economy and social make-up mean that the countryside is not uniform in social characteristics. Greater differences exist between rural areas than between rural and urban areas. Lives in small mining villages, towns of the former textile industry, small fishing villages now unable to find sufficient fish, hamlets of tied cottages of farm labourers, small council housing estates of rural district councils constructed seventy or eighty years ago, have greater differences than similarities. Nor do those who live there have much in common with those who own second homes, or work 30 miles away in a large city, or who have moved to a village location to get away from urbanised lifestyles. This newly arrived population may in fact hold traditional ideas of what the countryside should look like and be as vociferous as any in opposing changes in land use or approving low-cost housing schemes, introducing yet another element of social polarisation (Pugh 2003: 72).

EXCLUSION AND DISADVANTAGE IN THE COUNTRYSIDE

Policies to tackle social exclusion, from 1997 on, developed first within the context of urban disadvantage. Area-based projects such as the New Deal for Communities, Health Action Zones, Sure Start local programmes, community safety and crime reduction partnerships, community cohesion, and neighbourhood renewal were generated by policy action teams essentially responding to the concentration of exclusion in Britain's cities. Factors such as cost-effectiveness of programmes, targeting large numbers of the excluded and the hope of delivering quick, measurable outcomes persuaded government to begin there. Constraints on providing rural services were generally overlooked and continue to include the following:

- Public transportation is limited – 75 per cent of rural parishes have no daily bus service.
- Forty per cent have no shop or post office (70 per cent have no general store).
- Eighty per cent have no general practitioners.
- Fifty per cent have no school.
- There is a shortage of affordable housing, with young people finding it difficult to find entry-level housing.

The face of exclusion in rural areas

Disadvantage in rural areas is dispersed, mirroring the less dense population and geographical remoteness. Unlike major urban contexts where those with similar income levels tend to cluster together, people with very different levels of wealth live in close proximity to each other. Families on low income may be living next door to owners of a second home; social housing may exist across the street from large owner-occupied houses; those who have to take the bus may live near but are distinct from those who have multiple car ownership. As a consequence, social exclusion in sparse rural areas can feel like an individual, private matter. In less sparse areas there may be identifiable small pockets of poverty and some of these may even fall within the top fifth of most deprived areas in Britain but are still too small an area to fall within regeneration programmes tackling neighbourhood disadvantage (Shucksmith 2000: 39).

As a phenomenon, then, social exclusion in the countryside is more difficult to identify. In urban areas exclusion can be collectively experienced by people living in proximity – they are more visibly 'people in the same boat' – in a way that it is not in rural areas. As Shucksmith (2002: 39) puts it, in rural areas, 'neighbours often do not share the same experiences and poor rural households have little or no means to join forces in order to campaign for a better future'. Nor are rural communities autonomous, free-standing units; their degree of integration into the global economy, stability of the economy and proximity to metropolitan areas all impact on a community's capacity to resolve social problems (Reimer 2006).

There is, then, growing recognition that the countryside has its own patterns of disadvantage, inequality and exclusion that require action as part of a wider strategy for the countryside. A succession of government policy statements from 2000 on urged bringing services closer to local people, through improved accessibility and coordination, devolution and decentralisation. The creation of the Countryside Agency* aimed to improve rural environments and the Agency began to reformulate conceptions of rural exclusion in its landmark report *Pockets of Deprivation: Rural Initiative* (Countryside Agency 2003).

In the wake of this report, government pledged a rural dimension in reporting its annual appraisal of progress on tackling exclusion, *Opportunity for All*, and to introduce into its indices of multiple deprivation criteria more applicable to rural settings. Devolution of governmental power in 1998 to the three more rural nations of the United Kingdom – Wales, Scotland, and Northern Ireland – also encouraged greater attention to rural affairs on the part of central government. (In terms of land area Scotland is 95 per cent rural, and one of the major political parties, the Scottish National Party, has major strength in the countryside, ensuring greater visibility in policy development in that country.) Funded research began to enquire into the extent of social exclusion in rural areas – in Scotland, in Northern Ireland and in the upland farming areas of Wales and England where centuries of viable small farming households were suddenly in jeopardy. More specific investigations were also begun looking at the consequences of pit closures on mining villages, the experience of those with HIV and the pressures on lone parents in rural areas (see for example Hughes n.d., and Bennett *et al.* 2000).

---

*In 2008 parts of the Countryside Agency merged with Natural England and parts of the Commission for Rural Communities. The CRC was itself wound up by the Coalition government in 2010.

The extent of social exclusion in rural areas

Social exclusion in rural Britain is characterised by four groups: (i) older people living alone (predominantly widows) and older couples, often relying solely on the state pension – by far the largest single excluded group; (ii) children, especially of lone parents, or of households where no parent is working; (iii) young people, who often have to migrate great distances for work or higher education; (iv) low-paid, manual workers (rural areas contain a disproportionate number of people in low-wage sectors, notably agriculture and tourism, and in small workplaces).

Collectively they face higher costs than urban counterparts for certain basic necessities such as transportation, food and heating. Distance and remoteness play an important part in this. For example in the Western Isles in Scotland food takes on average nearly 25 per cent of a household budget, over twice the UK national average. Housing and fuel together also cost twice as much. There is heavier reliance on pensions and less inclination among local people to give personal financial information in order to pursue a claim for benefits (Rural Poverty and Inclusion Working Group 2001). Yet the small scale and nature of rural communities makes it difficult to target services or resources at specific social groups.

OLDER PEOPLE AND RURAL POVERTY

Poverty in general is less immediately visible in rural areas than in urban areas. The 'normalisation' of low income by disadvantaged older people, their careful management of household finances and their low expectations in terms of living standards are part of this. A sense of self-sufficiency, of not seeking additional support from the state and relying on help from informal sources, is a broad consequence. Mirroring the inequality elsewhere, 32 per cent of older-person households in rural Wales were living in poverty, predominantly among those who had lived in their area for thirty years or more, while newer arrivals had far higher incomes. On the other hand over 90 per cent of those living in poor households stated that they were 'very satisfied' or 'satisfied' with their area as a place to live, while only 6 per cent made any negative assessment (Milbourne and Doheny 2012).

THE FRAGMENTATION OF RURAL SERVICES: 'NO ONE IS IN CHARGE'

From the late 1980s on, government has sought to remove itself from providing services and instead to lay responsibility for that provision across partnerships involving both public and community voluntary organisations. This re-orientation has had a profound impact on rural life. Direct services from local authorities had once guaranteed the delivery of uneconomic services to more remote areas. Now local authorities no longer lead in service development or coordinate provision in the way that they once did, and instead we find a whole host of agencies involved in rural governance, drawn from the public, private and voluntary sectors. The countryside has been peculiarly vulnerable to the changes in those services.

First, the concepts of new public management and the separation of service providers from purchasers, the targeting of resources at identifiable groups of users most in need, and performance measurement all have built into them a bias tilting services toward dense urban settings and leaving rural areas without cover. Fire, ambulance, police and hospital services have been consolidated over wide geographical areas, and are no longer located in identifiable geographical communities. This consolidation has especially affected emergency and out-of-hours services, leaving rural populations feeling more insecure.

Second, creating competitive markets for services has often meant the thinning or withdrawal of all service provision in rural areas. For highly populated urban environments the resulting gaps in services were more easily filled by the voluntary or private sector (to a certain extent). For dispersed rural environments, however, this requires staffing day centres and youth centres, for example, either on a completely voluntary basis or around a part-time salaried post that itself has to rely on a staff of volunteers. And if they are to survive it leaves small, fledgling voluntary and local community organisations applying for grants, stretching their resources in time and knowledge even further.

Third, successive reorganisation of political jurisdictions often means that sustaining existing services, for example youth services or parent support initiatives, in rural areas is put on hold or overlooked. The combined effect of these three factors has led Shucksmith (2002) to call it a 'nobody-in-charge-world'.

CASE STUDY: OUT-OF-HOURS HEALTH CARE

For decades residents of a small town in a well-off shire county were able to contact a general practitioner from their local practice out of hours – from 6 pm in the evening to 8 am the following morning – by ringing the local surgery and getting the number of the GP on call for that night. Some years ago that service was replaced by a pool of out-of-hours GPs not connected with the local practice but available for consultation in the event of an emergency at a local cottage hospital some 5 miles away. A year ago that service in turn was abruptly suspended and replaced with a telephone consultation with a GP. There is still the possibility of a face-to-face consultation in the direst emergency but the distance to drive for that is some 25 miles.

REFLECT AND DECIDE: WHAT ARE THE BARRIERS?

Assume that parents suspect one of their twin daughters aged 10 may have contracted measles, despite having been vaccinated; she has awoken in the middle of the night, is hot and has a red rash on her stomach. Assume further that they live in the area described in the case study above. List the factors that they would need to have in place to make the 25-mile trip for a consultation at 3 am.

A special issue: accessibility of services and transport

Transport is both a vital resource and the source of social divide. Who has access to transport and in what form are major questions for social policy. While increased car ownership has brought benefits for the majority in rural areas, allowing longer-distance commuting and the maintenance of personal social networks across large areas, it has also reduced the customer base for those reliant on public transport. In 2012, 11 per cent of all rural households did not have a car, but this rose to 28 per cent for the bottom fifth of the population in income. For these households, journeys to work or access to services are constrained by limitations of public transport provision in low-density rural areas (DEFRA 2014).

In 2012, 46 per cent of households in most rural areas had a regular bus service close by (compared to 96 per cent of urban households) according to DEFRA – but 'regular' can mean virtually anything as long as the service is scheduled, even if no more than once a week (DEFRA 2014). Commuting by bus to work or for appointments can be difficult as rural services may not start early enough in a particular pick-up point or return late enough for a full working day. Lack of punctuality, cancellations and the 'original sin' of departing a pick-up point ahead of schedule are all familiar to the regular rural bus user.

Low mobility, in all its forms, plays a large role in social exclusion and particularly so in the countryside. The spate of recent research on transport and social exclusion in rural areas notes the following:

- Geographical isolation: dispersed locations may limit the ability to carry out activities in the immediate area while the growing popularity of centralised shopping and services excludes those without access to transport.
- Economic exclusion: problems with physical access and travel costs can limit access to higher education as well as the ability to find gainful employment.
- Time-based exclusion: juggling multiple responsibilities, especially for carers or lone parents, can result in high levels of time poverty.
- Fear-based exclusion: some people may feel threatened or vulnerable in particular areas.
- Space exclusion: some security and space-management strategies discourage socially excluded individuals from using certain public or semi-private spaces such as gated housing communities.

(adapted from Delbosc and Currie 2011 and Kenyon 2011)

One of the principal research conclusions is that social exclusion in the countryside is not due to a lack of social opportunities so much as a lack of *access* to those opportunities. In order to avoid social exclusion an individual requires a set of accessible facilities and social contacts. Some of these will be near enough so that transport times and costs are immaterial, while others will be more distant, meaning that transport and the money to pay for it is all-important. Exclusion can only be overcome then by: (i) promoting 'near-enough' social contacts, for example through policies increasing 'neighbourliness'; (ii) decentralising facilities and services; and (iii) reducing transport costs at the same time as increasing regularity of provision (Preston and Rajé 2007: 153).

The withdrawal of services has been matched by the shutting down of informal points of social contact. The wave of closures of primary schools, chapels, public houses, post offices, local constabularies and banks has fused with closed community hospitals, health clinics and doctors' surgeries (particularly out-of-hours services). Changes in the housing market and labour market have particularly affected young people, older people and women, who tend to have the fewest options in dealing with these widespread trends. These impediments to inclusion were closely bound up with failings of private and public services, most notably transport, social housing and child care. Migration and the loss of young people further ruptured informal support networks leaving older people socially isolated.

THE POWER OF PLACE

Hill farming (or 'upland' farming) in places like Northumberland, North Yorkshire, Cumbria, and Dartmoor covers some 18 per cent of the English countryside, with even greater percentages in Wales and Scotland. The natural beauty of the landscape hides adverse social and economic trends that have accelerated since 2005 when subsidy arrangements were dramatically altered and geared to acreage and not numbers of sheep. Hill farming has become a rapidly ageing occupation with the average age of farmers now over 60. Many live below the poverty line, earning less than farm labourers and well below the minimum wage. Villages are not only losing their young people but have fewer children in them to lose as they grow up. A preliminary report from the Commission for Rural Communities has noted the extent of 'increased stress, depression, poor health and a sense of isolation' (cited in Hetherington 2009). To draw on an urban metaphor, upland farming is a factory for social exclusion.

REFLECT AND DECIDE: HILL FARMING IN THE SOUTHWEST

A team at Exeter University has looked hard at the financing of hill farming in the southwest of England. Their study concluded that 44 per cent of the total output is in fact subsidised by the European Union's Common Agricultural Policy and is therefore wholly dependent on public funding – yet margins are 'hopelessly in the red' with incomes on average of just over £9,000 per annum. There are those who argue that this extensive subsidy should be put into other rural businesses and that hill farmers should be paid to leave their farms.

Do you think: (a) subsidies should be increased in order to raise standards of living; (b) left as they are; or (c) phased out and hill farmers paid for leaving their farms and finding work elsewhere? What would be the consequences of each option?

CASE STUDY: SMALL FAMILY FARMS IN NORTHERN IRELAND

Small farmers in Northern Ireland face parallel problems where, it is estimated, income from the agricultural sector has fallen by 80 per cent in real terms since 1995 (Heenan 2006). As with upland farming the economic viability of family farming is under threat but it continues because of the commitment to the way of life and the tradition of family land ownership which goes back generations, even as their children go elsewhere. In 2004 over 50 per cent of farmers in Northern Ireland were over 55 years old.

In the face of extreme economic disadvantage these farming communities retained the capacity to 'soldier on' and to 'suffer in silence' which they associated with strength of character. Mental health problems were generally kept hidden. Heenan has suggested that rural dwellers have more negative attitudes to mental illness than town dwellers, and among the farmers in County Down she found that mental illness was stigmatised and associated with weakness and shame. As one woman told her, the prevailing attitudes and norms meant there was little acknowledgement or understanding of mental health issues: 'Here it is all bottled up. You have problems but you don't talk about them. You are just expected to get on with it' (Heenan 2006).

In her study Heenan showed that access to health and social care among the farming families of County Down was influenced by economic, geographical, cultural and environmental factors, including the population's prevalent beliefs, expectations, attitudes and personal experiences of health and social care. Distinctive needs had combined with generations of experiences and attitudes to create particular challenges to those designing and delivering services. Heenan provided compelling evidence that on the one hand needs are greater in those areas where people had farmed on their own for generations, but on the other hand precisely those same areas had lost support services following the centralisation of services and closure of cottage hospitals. Her conclusion is that if service development and access strategies are to be successful, they must be underpinned by a clear understanding of service users' perspectives and attitudes (Heenan 2006).

SERVICE PROVISION IN RURAL AREAS

Social work in rural areas has generally followed what has been described as 'rural generalism' (Turbett 2006) which tended to reflect what was perceived as the communal elements of smaller towns and villages. Collier (2006: 42–43) observed that 'The generalist invents holistic ways to solve problems through refusal to be bound by disciplines or narrow job specifications. In rural areas such limitations almost always prove counter-productive.' The generalist model tended to harness the virtues of living and working within smaller face-to-face communities, relying on the capacity to cross professional boundaries easily and invoking community development models as a means for providing services.

Yet, as Turbett has shown, the rural generalist and community-oriented practice has found it difficult to survive in the face of powerful trends toward specialisation and statutory procedural frameworks taking place at national level, though he noted continued efforts of practitioners in Scotland to maintain a community orientation and provide flexible responses to user need (Turbett 2006).

Tackling social exclusion in rural areas will in practice follow many of the same approaches as in urban-based social work. A child in need, a care leaver, a young person not in education, employment or training will have the same compelling case for services as if they were from an urban neighbourhood. But in providing these the practitioner faces a different set of forces that shape that practice.

Linking community development and social care

The exclusion of adult service users can in part be overcome by linking the objectives of social care with those of community development. They are in fact strongly complementary. The requirements for tackling social exclusion – partnerships, local approaches, community engagement and anti-poverty strategies – are also important elements in community and neighbourhood development. The Scottish government, Welsh Assembly and Commission for Rural Communities (CRC) in England have all pushed hard to tackle social exclusion in rural areas through community development (Welsh Assembly 2004; Scottish Executive 2001; CRC 2008).

As Barr and his colleagues have asserted: 'Methods of community development can help achieve the objectives of progressive community care, whilst engagement with user communities helps community development to realise its vision of inclusiveness' (Barr *et al.* 2001). A community development framework places social care services and user involvement in a different light. People are motivated to learn, not by the invitation to join a consultation process for existing services but by the desire to solve real problems that beset them and their locality. Learning effective skills and understanding the process of practical action becomes a powerful form of education.

Community development approaches to social care focus on bending resources and power towards disadvantaged neighbourhoods where there are likely to be large numbers of people in need of care. Groups of care users may form communities of interest through their common experiences and needs that prompt them to act on a collective basis. Much of community care is based on the premise that users should be able to participate as fully as they are able; the task of community development is to help develop this participation. The principles of 'normalisation' and citizenship cannot be achieved without the active participation of care groups in the planning, provision and consumption of care services (Barr *et al.* 1997: 3).

Social care practitioners need several skills to fuse their work with community development. They need to engage with people in the community in setting aims and objectives. For example, in the setting-up of a carers' support scheme in a neighbourhood by a social worker with older people, consulting the community by advertising and holding a public meeting in the time-honoured way would likely have a poor response. It is more effective for practitioners to identify ways in which they are already in touch with members of the community through home-care services, low-cost day centres, lunch clubs or contacts with family and relatives. This allows them to pool useful information, to find articulate spokespeople for their interests and engage in lateral thinking around others' ideas. It also initiates discussion with potential partner services such as health visitors, general practitioners and voluntary agencies.

CASE STUDY: VILLAGE AGENTS

The Village agents scheme provides support and information to older people in rural areas where a lack of available counselling is evident. The Village agent concept was first identified as a recommendation from the Department for Work and Pension's research on rurality in 2002/3 which confirmed that a high percentage of rural residents would be happy approaching someone they knew and trusted within the community for help.

The schemes, run by rural community councils, cover the more isolated parishes as a bridge between local community and statutory and voluntary organisations; agents provide information (but not advice), promote access to services, and identify unmet needs within their community. Support is provided across a wide range of areas, including health, social care, personal safety, fuel poverty and benefits/pensions. Although help and support are offered to any disadvantaged and isolated person, the agents predominantly work with older people in their seventies and eighties. Village agents are recruited locally from a range of backgrounds including former Citizens Advice Bureau employees, counsellors, and some without direct experience or qualifications.

(adapted from CRC 2008)

Living and working in the same place: implications for practice

There are challenges for practitioners who live in the very communities they serve. Face-to-face familiarity and the tracking of people's movements in work and out means that professional roles (of doctors, lawyers, social workers) overlap with face-to-face contacts that occur outside of those roles. This blurs public and private knowledge and communication, with service users often holding concrete information on the personal lives of professionals – where they live, phone number, marriage status, their children. As Pugh writes: 'Workers who wish to maintain a professional "distance", or even mistakenly some sense of "mystique", may find it difficult to do this because their "otherness" and professional power may visibly be seen not to extend to other aspects of their context' (Pugh 2007: 75).

This lack of anonymity raises issues of privacy and confidentiality – and how they are tackled. Some of the qualities affecting rural social work (lack of anonymity) are based on the assumption of stable, long-standing communities where information about individuals passes quickly from person to person. HIV sufferers for example in such a context may be reluctant to seek medical help. But there are considerable variations in types of rural communities – some are stable, others not; even the most stable are prone to movement and reconstitution. For example the postman/woman who knows many people, even down to the receipt of particular letters, may themselves fall to the rapid changes in the postal service. (Of course cities are no longer a place where a person can lose themselves either; extensive surveillance in cities through CCTV and automatic modes for web and email surveillance may well prove more intrusive for urban residents than word-of-mouth information for rural individuals.)

REFLECT AND DECIDE: BOYS IN YOUR GARDEN

A social worker lives in a small town where she runs a small, all-volunteer youth centre for young people between the ages of 13 and 17. One day she came in from work to find rubbish strewn all around the garden – tell-tale signs of empty pop bottles, sweet wrappers, cigarette packs. That night, starting at 4 am in the morning, she received a series of phone calls with weird, put-on voices asking for different individuals by name and accompanied by some fits of laughter. Although most of the callers had their numbers withheld, one or two did not and she was able to identify these as belonging to two of the young people who attended the centre and who she knew were living right around the corner.

Would you report these events to the police? Go to the parents of the young people who you knew had made the phone calls? Talk to the young people themselves when you next encountered them? Say or do nothing on the assumption that the behaviour was out of character and was unlikely to happen again? Make a list of the pros and cons of each of these responses to the situation.

REFLECT AND DECIDE: A RURAL CHILDREN'S CENTRE

A rural children's centre, based in a small town some 10 miles from the city, delivers services over a wide area in the borough. Two staff, both female, hold clinics in smaller towns and villages offering guidance on breast feeding and stimulating children's development for parents who drop in. Other staff provide a family café in the same locations where they offer advice and reassurance to young parents concerning a child's tantrums or eating healthy foods. In addition the centre funds St John Ambulance to put on a series of first-aid training sessions, 'Baby Safe', that teach parents of new-born infants what to do if their infant should have an accident or suffer some other physical emergency.

The centre delivers its programme in small halls and youth centres. The resources to provide the advice session on breast feeding alone are as follows:

- Time required to drive from the centre and back: 1 hour × 2 staff members.
- Expenses claim for car mileage: 18 miles.
- Time staffing the advice session: 2 hours.

The service also relies on local volunteers to open and close the youth centre in which the sessions take place. If you were manager of this service how many mothers would you want to see attending the advice sessions to justify the resources used?

CASE STUDY: TRANSPORT IN COUNTY DOWN

The would-be health service users that Deirdre Heenan talked to mentioned the lack of transport as the chief barrier to practice. She reported that there was only one daily bus service from the study area into the local town. As she wrote,

> This bus was a 'school run' and left at 8.30 am and returned at 3.30 pm, and there was no service during the school holidays in July and August. There were no community transport schemes and no special provision for the rural area. Twenty-two of those interviewed were entitled to a free bus-pass (being over 65 years of age), but only one had applied for the pass; the others simply regarded it as a waste of time. As one said, 'It's a joke when you think about it, a free bus-pass but no bus'.
> (Heenan 2006: 382)

She concluded that free public transport is meaningless in a rural area where there is scant public transport in the first place. In towns social services would organise bus transport to services; in the country people are expected to organise their own. Services never come to them; 'the onus is always on them to get there'.

CASE STUDY: BENEFIT TAKE-UP SCHEME IN A RURAL AREA

Powys County Council, covering a large rural area in mid-Wales, uses workers based at home who take initial referrals, by phone or secure website, for those needing welfare advice. When giving face to face advice, or when they need to do administrative work, they are able to travel to designated venues and referral agencies where facilities for administrative work or meeting users is available.

Forming partnerships in rural areas

Working in rural areas, especially if full-time, can be an isolating experience. Recognising that this applies to all service practitioners, workers need to take a more proactive stance in articulating a need for a particular service development, promoting partnerships for specific initiatives. If not, quite likely the rural dimension will go by default, as pressing claims – both political through the service hierarchy and from service users and perhaps local media – will force attention back to urban-based problems.

In large geographical areas with dispersed populations, supervision and peer contact may be patchy. It is likely that there will be few or no co-workers on hand and line management may well be miles away. Specialist knowledge will be hard won – based on what the worker has accumulated on their own.

Ellis (2002) explains how social exclusion happens as a matter of course even when service organisations are trying to engage rural communities. She notes that they will (i) presume levels of skills and community energy that are not necessarily there, and (ii) overlook the displacement of existing community groups through their mobilisation and enrolment of individuals. Her research suggests policy making has been naive in assuming that bottom-up rural development will necessarily lead to more extensive local participation. Rather her study shows that even bottom-up development will be controlled and shaped by external gatekeepers, and will almost in spite of itself serve the needs and interests of the more powerful sections of the rural population – unless practice becomes sensitive to processes of exclusion and power relations in rural society.

Participation has its costs in time and money and some rural social strata can bear these costs more easily than others. Gentrification for example has brought with it a new franchise of middle-class suburbanites that has recomposed the rural class structure along with restructuring the local property market. Along with this comes an accumulated set of interests, resources, affiliations and cultural resources that are assertive, active, and familiar with the language and mechanics of organisations and adept at framing points of view tailored to that. The effect of gentrification is not only to displace lower-income households in the housing market but also to raise the social, psychic and economic costs of participation for those who can ill afford them.

EXCLUDED GROUPS IN THE COUNTRYSIDE

Difficulties facing young people in rural areas

The older teenagers who spoke to Glendinning et al. (2008) about their social lives, family and social networks, and their community, noted these as both close-knit and caring and as intrusive and controlling. Surprisingly it was evident that community links were important to young people's sense of wellbeing, but getting the balance right between intrusiveness and support and attachment was difficult. This is particularly true of young women who often lack a social and geographical space where they can associate and which they can identify as their own. Young people are highly visible in their communities, and subject to adult scrutiny and in many cases disapproval, viewed as a problem rather than as contributory members of their communities.

Dealing with this scrutiny is not easy. Marginalisation also arises from being denied one's own space for social interaction, not because of physical distance and lack of transport but as a result of power-laden interactions with peers and adults within the village. 'For rural youth, marginality is in part founded upon adult surveillance and regulation of activities and spaces within the countryside' (Leyshon 2003: 236, cited in Shucksmith 2004).

Gender is a key dimension affecting young people's feelings about their communities with significant implications for sense of wellbeing and out-migration. Young men drinking in village pubs gain affirmation of their rural identity from peers and older males by adopting an exclusive, hierarchical, homophobic and sexist discourse that serves to marginalise young women and other young men whose identity as 'rural' is thereby called into question (Shucksmith 2004: 3).

In the transition to adulthood and particularly in finding a place in the labour market further difficult choices await young people in rural areas. They tend to become integrated into one of 'two quite separate labour markets – the national (distant, well-paid, with career opportunities) and the local (poorly paid, insecure, unrewarding and with fewer prospects)'. Social class and education are two major determinants – as they are in urban Britain – that give some young people access to national job opportunities. Significantly for those whose lack of educational credentials confine them to local labour markets, further education and training are much less available than for their counterparts in towns, and their life chances correspondingly reduced (Shucksmith 2000: 4).

A range of factors associated with rural school systems further hobble work to tackle the social exclusion of young people:

- insufficient resources to recruit and retain specialist staff around important resources such as special educational needs (SEN), English as an additional language and pastoral support;
- a lack of alternative provision for excluded pupils owing to travelling distances;
- a lack of employer engagement and inconsistent or patchy provision across institutions of the 14–19 Diploma programme;
- insufficient availability of apprenticeships and an almost complete lack of GCSE evening classes outside major towns, making it impossible for poor rural households to gain or improve their qualifications once they have left school.

The development of youth services provides a good example of the shrinking role of the local authority in service provision. In the mid-1970s, county youth federations offered widespread funding for local youth services in rural and urban areas. There was a system of training volunteers at local colleges who could gain entry-level qualifications for youth work as well as opportunities for observation and mentoring at other youth clubs. To assist smaller clubs a roster of staff was available to underpin the work at local clubs.

These once robust federations are a pale shadow of their former selves, employing far fewer staff who are confined largely to supplying training, a trend that has only accelerated after the youth service was, first, subsumed by Connexions, the youth advisory organisation, and then, after Connexions itself was abolished, either contracted out, picked up by voluntary organisations or – more likely – disappeared altogether.

The activities of extended schools mean that schools too are competing to host activities in order to show how their facilities are used by the community and after hours. In rural schools young people's friendship groups may be distributed over wide catchment areas and may be further undermined at sixth form as the choice to attend a sixth form college becomes available. The means of transport for young people rests wholly on parents' driving, or on a patchy bus service. Understandably young people are eager to learn to drive themselves and to acquire their own vehicle. Driving competence becomes an essential skill since 'bridging' contacts that enable young people to move to higher or further education or the job market are built on their own resources and not least on the capacity to drive. Poverty and inequality makes a mark here too: the cost of insurance for a young driver is beyond low-income families.

Working with lone parents in rural areas

The number of lone parents in specific rural areas can reach over 8 per cent of all households. Rural lone parents are more likely to have become so through marriage breakdown (as opposed to breakdown of non-married partnership or never partnered);

more likely to experience geographical relocation; and more likely to receive maintenance for children from former partners.

Earlier research had highlighted lower levels of labour market participation among rural women, in general stemming from a lack of expectation of obtaining secure employment as well as giving priority to a domestic and caring role. There were reasons for this choice: jobs in rural areas are low-wage and insecure with no sick pay or paid leave. It is also more difficult to find employers who are prepared to work around school hours – many remain 'unenlightened' about work–life balance. The likely work would be administrative positions and clerical jobs, such as school secretaries, receptionists and office clerks, and personal service work such as care assistants in nursing homes, learning support workers, teaching assistants and carers for adults and children with learning disabilities.

The dilemmas facing lone parents in rural areas in regard to work are similar to those all parents face, as discussed in Chapter 4, but compounded by the limits of the rural labour market. Hughes (2004) noted that there was little correlation between age of children and number of children and the decision to take on paid work, but the ill health of children had a profound effect on the decision of lone parents. In the rural areas she studied she found that day-care centres would not take disabled children since care for the disabled child is more expensive: it is labour-intensive and expertise is difficult to find. In general those without educational qualifications were less likely to be in work than those with a qualification by a ratio of 2 to 1. Mothers saw the working tax credit as a major boost in supporting low incomes since child maintenance is disregarded.

KEY POINTS

❑   The countryside is changing rapidly as agriculture loses its dominant position, young people leave and a more affluent middle class moves in.

❑   Social exclusion affects a large proportion of those living in rural areas but it is more dispersed and less readily 'visible'. Many of the government's programmes for tackling social exclusion were intended for disadvantaged urban areas and were field tested there. They have not transferred to rural areas easily.

❑   The national trend towards separating purchasers of services from the providers, and towards delivering services through broad partnerships involving public and voluntary sector agencies, has had the effect of thinning out services to rural areas. Statutory services which once underpinned a guarantee of provision have withdrawn from rural areas.

❑   The plight of hill farming families, lone parents, young people and older people in rural areas is multi-dimensional, with certain costs – for transport and food in particular – weighing on the budgets of those on low income.

KEY READING

Colin Turbett, *Rural Social Work Practice in Scotland* (British Association of Social Workers, 2010).

James Garo Derounian, 'Now you see it . . . now you don't: a review of rural community organizing in England', Third Sector Research Centre Working Paper 116.

CHAPTER 9

RACISM AND SOCIAL EXCLUSION

THIS CHAPTER COVERS

- Exclusionary effects of racism.

- The concept of institutional racism and its implications for practice.

- Ways in which practitioners can combat racism such as anti-bias work with children and young people.

- Links between racism and asylum seekers.

- How practitioners can develop a practice to advance community cohesion.

This chapter highlights the role that racism plays in underpinning the social exclusion of different ethnic groups in Britain and looks at ways that its damage can be overcome in practice. Within this broad objective it seeks to do two things: (i) to examine the way racism has adopted hidden coded expressions; and (ii) to look more closely at what integration and multiculturalism – the overcoming of racism – mean.

Social exclusion, as used generically by government, has been criticised as 'colour blind' since it often ignores ethnic difference (Parekh 2000: 82). Yet ethnic difference is a powerful determinant of exclusion, and racism, the mass intimidation of a people based on their skin colour, even more so. Racism is not singular but plural. 'There are', writes Tariq Modood, 'colour or phenotype racisms but there are also cultural racisms which build on "colour" a set of antagonistic or demeaning stereotypes based on allied or real cultural traits' (Modood 2007: 44–45). Islamophobia for example is as much about 'race' as it is about faith.

Disadvantage and social exclusion among minority ethnic groups

Disadvantage and social exclusion dominate many minority ethnic communities and racism has a good deal to do with this. Ethnic minorities in England are more likely to live in deprived neighbourhoods than the White British majority: 46 per cent of Bangladeshis and a third of Pakistanis live in such neighbourhoods, higher than any other ethnic group, reflecting income-deprived neighbourhoods, depleted living environments, and poor services. That percentage however is a reduction on the 2001 census.

The unemployment rate of ethnic minorities is almost twice that of the White British population. Disparities in employment are greatest for Black ethnic groups compared with the White British majority. One explanation for this is labour market discrimination compounded by disadvantages in relation to education, health and housing (Jivraj and Khan 2013).

Mumtaz Lalani and colleagues carried out research in Glasgow, Leicester and Luton on the effects of segregation for African Caribbean, Indian and Pakistani residents. They found:

- Racism in education and employment varies by locality, contributing to differences in outcome according to neighbourhood.
- Social segregation severely limits knowledge of education and labour market systems and how to negotiate them – which in turn affects job finding. Self-employment – with labour limited to the family – deepens social segregation and in some communities reinforces norms of the woman's role as nurturer rather than breadwinner.
- Education, careers guidance and employment services vary enormously and with varying access to them. They may or may not be tailored to reflect the diversity of ethnicities in a locality.

(Lalani *et al.* 2014)

The recession and its after-effects hit minority ethnic groups hard. Between 2012 and 2013, unemployment levels for the UK as a whole and for white ethnic groups remained constant – at 8 and 7 per cent respectively – while unemployment among minority ethnic groups rose from 13 to 14 per cent. The rise was particularly noticeable among Black ethnic groups (up from 16 to 17 per cent) and Pakistani/Bangladeshi ethnic groups (from 17 to 19 per cent). In 2014, 16–24-year-olds from minority ethnic backgrounds had an unemployment rate of 37 per cent, up from 33 per cent in 2012. For the UK as a whole, unemployment in this age group was 21 per cent and had been constant for the past three years (Chalabi 2014).

UNDERSTANDING 'RACE' AND RACISM

'Race' is a bogus concept, nineteenth-century in origin, deployed to suggest a sense of inherent physical and cognitive superiority and inferiority among different peoples. It is a purely social construct without biological foundation which is why most writers now use the term in inverted commas. The paradox lies in the fact that on the basis of this false concept there are nevertheless groups and individuals who use it to justify overt discrimination, prejudice, violence and hate crimes. In short, there is racism though 'race' does not exist.

Gadd and Dixon (2011: 43) argue that the very 'emptiness' of race as a social category accounts for its destructiveness because it 'enables its signifiers – colour, face shape, hair and increasingly religion, language, nationality and citizenship – to become invested with the kinds of feelings about which people are most uncomfortable – anxiety, inadequacy, envy and guilt'. As a consequence, 'race' is a term ripe for polarisation and binary thinking, splitting objects into the loved and the hated and confusing self and object as projective identification dominates.

Much sociological work on racism tends to predict too much racism among certain sections of the working class and too little in other, less deprived sections of society. It overlooks the tolerant resident in a housing estate and links racism to native sense of being deprived. Gadd and Dixon instead put forward the idea of the 'contradictory racist subject' – sometimes bigoted, sometimes tolerant and occasionally able to identify across social differences – but vulnerable to change of attitude when crises occur (ibid.).

Racist concepts and the hate movements founded on them fuel the mass intimidation of, and violence against, designated groups of people such as asylum seekers, Roma travellers, immigrants and refugees. The civil disturbances in northern cities such as Oldham and Bradford in 2001 were in the main conducted along ethnic lines fuelled by white antagonism to perceived injustices as well as by the gulf of separation between different communities. The more recent electoral success of UKIP is based in part on resentment toward new arrivals, particularly in England's seaside towns, but has spread as fears of immigration, particularly from within the European Union, have been heightened by government and media. It is another strong indicator that racism and its coded accessories are still a powerful influence and remain the major agent of intolerance.

DEFINING 'RACE' AND RACISM

'Race' appears as a biological and cultural construct to classify one group of people from another, using such criteria as skin colour, language or customary behaviour. It is also used to denote status and lineage (Burke and Harrison 2001: 282). Racial and ethnic categories vary over time in meaning and importance. Generally they imply a distinction between 'whites' and other minorities of colour.

Racism 'consists of conduct or words or practices which disadvantage or advantage people because of their colour, culture, or ethnic origin. In its more subtle form it is as damaging as in its overt form' (Macpherson 1999: 20).

'Whiteness' refers to white people's favoured position in the social order relative to other racial groups. It describes the automatic, unmerited advantages and benefits conferred upon ownership of white skin by society. It does not mean that every white person is materially or otherwise more advantaged than Black or Asian people (Lawrence 2001).

INSTITUTIONAL RACISM

The concept of institutional racism was advanced in the Macpherson inquiry (Macpherson 1999) into the murder of a young black man, Stephen Lawrence, by a gang of white youths. It denotes the built-in tendency of services, especially the police, to not see the racialised dimensions of their own practice. It refers to policies and practices within and across institutions that produce outcomes that chronically favour a racial group and put other racial groups at a disadvantage. It reinforces a key pillar of exclusion by building a wall of suspicion and distance between a service essential for a sense of community safety – the police – and local residents. The focus of institutional racism is on the ways in which services and practices produce discriminatory results intentionally or unintentionally, and one of the great strengths of the Macpherson Report was that it required examination of the unintended consequences of the activity of public institutions and service agencies, and provides a new set of instruments with which to monitor and oppose racist activity of all kinds. The report defined a racist incident, for example, as 'any incident which is perceived to be racist by the victim or any other person' (Macpherson 1999: 328). Further, it made clear that all local government and relevant agencies and not just the police should adopt this standard. The subsequent Race Relations (Amendment) Act of 2000 did indeed make this standard mandatory for all public agencies to uphold.

Much of the criticism of the report at the time it was published centred on this subjective definition of what a racist incident is, which, critics said, meant that an allegation of racism was its own proof because in the view of the victim it had happened. This criticism has died away and the report remains a landmark in understanding the full nature of racism.

DEFINITION OF INSTITUTIONAL RACISM

Institutional racism is the collective failure of an organisation to provide an appropriate and professional service to people because of their colour, culture, or ethnic origin. It can be seen or detected in processes, attitudes and behaviour which amount to discrimination through unwitting prejudice, ignorance, thoughtlessness and racist stereotyping which disadvantage minority ethnic people (Macpherson 1999: para 6.34).

Institutional racism refers to characteristics of formal political, economic and organisation structures that generate racialised but nevertheless widely legitimised outcomes – outcomes that cannot be traced to obvious racial biases in the practices themselves or to acts of individual racism by staff or officials in these institutions. 'Nevertheless these institutions maintain cultures and practices that, in the end, disregard the particular needs of disadvantaged racial groups or facilitate unequal outcomes for different racial groups' (Lawrence 2001: 45).

The report also made a sustained attempt to see overturned the unwitting prejudice and thoughtless deployment of racist stereotypes embedded in the norms and values by which police officers defined their roles and the legitimacy of their activities. As

Lea (2000) observes, the report saw prejudice as something into which individuals are socialised. It is not the kind of contact between predominately white police and black people that is the issue, 'but rather the *lack of other contact outside that relationship*' (Lea 2000: 222, emphasis in the original).

There are those who argue that the concept is so broad that it is meaningless. But as Charles Blow has written, the deniers of institutional racism,

> or more precisely, its concealers – demand an articulated proof for something that moves in silence. They demand to see chapter and verse for something that is unwritten. They demand to know the names of the individual archi-tects of a structure built subconsciously over time by each member of the vast multitudes adding their own bit, like beavers adding branches to a dam.
>
> (Blow 2015)

Social work and institutional racism

Social work has long sought to overcome exclusion based on racism and to its great credit had tackled institutional racism well before the Macpherson Report. It was also among the very first professions to focus on racism as a means of exclusion and to make anti-racism central to its practice. From the late 1980s on, the old Central Council for Education and Training in Social Work (CCETSW) explicitly brought in a black perspective to its deliberations and worked out a set of competencies for anti-racist practice (CCETSW 1991). Sometimes these policies caused unease because of the Council's categorical and top-down approach (Penketh 2001). More important was the new thinking within social work in which 'race' was not viewed as 'essentialist', that is innately embodying fixed qualities whether positive or negative, but as a product of social relationships (Stone and Butler 2000).

The clear professional acknowledgement is that racism in public agencies is only eradicated through specific coordinated action within the agencies themselves and through social institutions at large – particularly schools, from pre-primary school upwards. Social work has much to contribute here through its involvement in early years work; anti-racism is foremost a matter of heart and mind and it begins in the early years (see below).

RACE RELATIONS (AMENDMENT) ACT 2000

The Race Relations (Amendment) Act 2000 embedded the major concepts of the Macpherson Report in statute by amending the Race Relations Act 1976 in two major ways:

- It extended the public's protection against racial discrimination by public authorities.
- It placed a new, enforceable, positive duty on public authorities not to engage in racial discrimination in any of its practices. This lays on each authority the urgent task of examining their practice to ensure that the forms of institutional and unwitting

racism, as much as the intentional racism of individual officers, are eliminated from their practice. While the Act applies formally only to public authorities it is also clearly intended to apply to private and voluntary organisations and other bodies such as multi-agency partnerships.

COMMUNITY COHESION

The concept of community cohesion provides an indirect way to tackle racism. The riots that occurred largely along ethnic divisions in several northern cities in the early 2000s shook both central and local government. They seemed to prefigure a Britain that was built on segregation and violent discord between south Asian communities, the police and some white communities. The sources of conflict as identified in the official inquiries that followed (Cantle 2008; Ousley 2001) stemmed from the consequences of communities living in isolation from one another. These investigations highlighted what they considered to be strong evidence of the extent of social exclusion arising from segregation of ethnic communities through separate housing, the lack of common leisure, recreational, sporting and cultural activities and schools dominated by a single culture or faith.* Policies for promoting community cohesion were rapidly assembled and proved remarkably durable. The National Action Plan on Social Inclusion defined community cohesion as a central aspect of its wider social inclusion agenda, suggesting that areas most at risk of community tensions are also those with high levels of social exclusion (Department of Work and Pensions 2005).

The aim was a wider sense of inclusion through reinforcing ideas of common citizenship, diversifying schools which by design or default were based on a single culture or faith, developing integrated housing schemes and instituting programmes to promote contact between faiths and ethnic groups. Whether such policies can achieve these objectives rests on the assumption that common principles and shared values can ultimately be found in a multi-ethnic and multi-faith society. Yet in diverse communities this is by no means certain and trying to prescribe certain outcomes, no matter how desirable, may have unintended consequences. As Madeleine Bunting has written:

> A comfortable multicultural society is . . . made on the street, in the school –
> in the myriads of relationships of friends, neighbours and colleagues. That's
> where new patterns of accommodation to bridge cultural differences are
> forged; that's where minds change, prejudices shift and alienation is eased.
> (Bunting 2006)

Community cohesion policies have attempted to deal with both elements of communal segregation: both trying to diminish spatial segregation – or what Briggs calls 'cure' strategies – and at the same time trying to soften the negative impact of segregation on social outcomes – what Briggs calls 'mitigate' strategies – without trying to change patterns of geographical residence (Briggs 2004).

---

*It is interesting to note that the origins of the riots in 2011 were seen differently – the product of bad parenting and troubled families.

Pursuing cohesion has significantly changed the orientation of the government's anti-racist strategies and to some extent has overshadowed the more radical perspectives of the Macpherson Report (Worley 2005). While continuing to promote respect for all cultures it now places greater weight on social integration and shared values, playing down both racism and economic deprivation as potent elements in community discourses (Worley 2005; McGhee 2003). The strong commitments to tackling institutional racism embodied in the Race Relations (Amendment) Act of 2000 have been downgraded.

The perceived dangers of segregation overlap with divisions between faith communities that are themselves entwined with ethnic and class divisions. Ted Cantle, author of the key report on the disturbances in 2001, has described these as 'layers of separation' – around language, education, use of leisure time, housing, lifestyle and familial and social structure (Cantle 2008). Awareness of how profound these divisions are has reawakened debate about the viability of multiculturalism. Multicultural definitions of citizenship, formed in the 1980s and 1990s and particularly embraced by the social work profession, acknowledged that different groups have different values, interests and needs and should enjoy rights of 'recognition' and respect. While there were problems with this approach, namely that it often ignored differences *within* particular cultures and overlooked the fluidity of boundaries between ethnic groups including White British, it nevertheless provided a framework of separate cultural rights as part of a larger mosaic of cultures. Now, in the wake of concepts of community cohesion, members of ethnic minorities (remembering of course that in many urban areas they are majorities) are facing a narrower definition of citizenship and being asked to adopt a set of shared national values.

Settled residents' attitudes to new arrivals: 'hunkering down' or informally tolerant?

The assertion that living in ethnically diverse areas undermines trust and community cohesion – both for newcomers and already settled residents of a locality – has been around a long time. Social science itself has had a long preoccupation with 'the stranger' and the immigrant seen as a force that disrupts the bonds of kinship and neighbourliness. Putnam's research for example linked the degree of ethnic diversity to the trust in neighbours among residents – the greater the diversity, the lower the general sense of trust (Putnam 2007).

The degree of trust among residents for one another is widely regarded as the 'social glue' essential to holding communities together, but it may of course be group-based, felt only *within* a particular social group, rather than across a neighbourhood or locality as a whole. In that case trust becomes something that is extended to or withheld from others based on group membership. Extending trust to another group means putting one's own group at risk, vulnerable to the behaviour of the group to whom that trust has been extended. Hence the caution that is often expressed between groups as to when and when not to exchange trust (Schmid *et al.* 2014: 666). Putnam argues that some ethnic groups 'hunker down' in ethnically diverse environments by withdrawing trust from others, including, eventually, those within their own ethnic groups (Putnam 2007).

This is an issue that is far from settled and Putnam's concept has its critics. Social psychologists have long noted that increased intergroup contact reduces the sense of threat between groups. Recent investigations in England show that the *indirect* effects of diversity through everyday contact between groups have a positive effect on all types of trust and attitudes for both 'in' and 'out' groups. Diversity offers opportunities for intergroup contact that reduces the sense of threat and fosters trust (Schmid *et al.* 2014: 672). It is segregation rather than diversity that negatively affects trust, as being able to see diverse individuals interacting positively with each other has the potential to 'rub off' on others – a form of tolerance. Other research has found that while settled residents could express concern regarding migration as a mass social movement, with real and symbolic consequences for their towns and cities, they also expressed tolerant and even favourable views toward the orderly behaviour of migrants as neighbours living along-side them (Griffiths 2014: 1123). Through small norms of courtesy and politeness, the social order in the studied locale – in this case Crewe in Cheshire – was managed and maintained through weak but '*civilised relationships*' between migrants and established residents, thus failing to culminate in conflict between the two groups (ibid.).

In Northern Ireland there is a difference between 'single identity' and 'cross-identity' approaches to community relations. Each is appropriate depending on objectives. Single identity approaches help individuals develop deeper understanding of culture and identity and self-awareness of a particular group *before* engaging in dialogue and exchanges with members of other groups. It is a useful approach par-ticularly when there exists a wider atmosphere of antagonism, or when there are risks to cross-community approaches or when the sense of identity may be relatively weak within particular groups (Kelly and Philpott 2003). An example in England is the 'Healing History' project in Mansfield, a predominantly white working-class town in the Midlands, which examined the once strong working-class culture that formed around the mining industry and the contemporary impact of that culture on attitudes towards race and minority ethnic groups after the mines had all closed (Cantle 2008: 203). On the other hand, such approaches may only encourage stereotyped views of one's own culture, creating 'better informed bigots' when the overriding aim should be to encourage greater critical self-awareness of culture and to enable individuals to understand what is positive and what is problematic in their beliefs and values. It should build in steps to enable members of a group to recognise how and why identi-ties are formed, to understand the notion of multiple identities and to recognise both similarities and differences with others (Kelly and Philpott 2003: 37).

Another useful distinction is between 'associational' and 'everyday' forms of cross-cultural networks. Associational networks are formed through relationships based on organisations and provide a strong element binding local civic and commercial life together, particularly between religious communities. Everyday networks on the other hand do not require organisations but are founded on individual relationships and are more prominent in rural areas. Cantle (2008: 190), in his explanation of the distinction between the two types, argues that associational networks provide a 'sturdier bulwark of peace'. In the conflict between Hindu and Muslim communities that he investigated, Varshney (2002) cited the pre-existing local networks of civic engagement between the two communities as the single most important factor in the maintenance of peace even in a period of heightened antagonism. Those networks facilitated communication, proved rumours false, and provided information to the local administration. Where such networks are missing communal identities lead to endemic violence.

Predominantly the work on community cohesion has been cross-cultural in several different fields, such as twinning schools that are dominated by one culture and encouraging mixed intakes, creating residential areas with mixed ethnicity, creating cross-cultural employment opportunities in public sector work and in policing and community safety (Cantle 2008: 206). 'Mono-cultural' schools – often faith-based – pose a particular difficulty. They are not intentionally acting as agents of social exclusion or deliberately drawing intakes from segregated residential patterns, but rather on what Cantle has called a 'critical mass' model where adherents of a particular faith are clustered in an area and the numbers become sufficiently large to establish strong local institutions. Interaction with other faiths and cultures takes place but within a context underpinned by its dominance. To be successful, school twinning schemes, such as those in Bradford and Oldham (where fifty schools are twinned), need to be buttressed by joint teaching programmes and shared extra-curricular activities, especially ones involving cross-community parental links (Cantle 2008: 221).

Full *integration* is only finally achieved when ethnic hierarchies have been eradicated; when equality of opportunity is equitably distributed between ethnic groups and where all such groups are encouraged to contribute to every aspect of society.

REFLECT AND DECIDE: AISA

Aisa is a community support worker for an early years project. Her parents came from Bangladesh some twelve years ago. They and Aisa are devout Muslims. Four members of the project are developing a model for 'women-centred practice'. Aisa notices that she has certain disagreements with some aspects of that model but keeps these to herself. At one meeting two of these colleagues begin talking about 'the mosque' in ways that Aisa regards as disrespectful and condescending; in particular, they underscore several times how men run the affairs of the mosque and are quite oppressive.

What should Aisa say at this point? Should she discuss the tone of the meeting with her parents? To whom should she turn for support? Should she begin to think about modifying her devotion?

REFUGEES, IMMIGRATION AND ASYLUM SEEKERS

Refugees and asylum seekers from Africa and the Middle East and new arrivals from Eastern Europe are among the most excluded groups in Britain. They often face similar experiences to those of ethnic minorities – dislocation, powerlessness and discrimination – while having to deal with major recent trauma and with fewer support systems to call on. Tension between new arrivals and the settled community is sometimes reported by local newspapers in ways that are often xenophobic and tacitly racist, such as those that announced the arrival of Polish and Romanian workers in the early years of the twenty-first century.

UN CONVENTION ON REFUGEES: DEFINITION AND MEANING

A refugee according to the Convention is someone who is unable or unwilling to return to their country of origin owing to a well-founded fear of being persecuted for reasons of race, religion, nationality, membership of a particular social group, or political opinion.

The Convention is a rights-based instrument underpinned by fundamental principles: Convention provisions are to be applied without discrimination as to race, religion or country of origin – or sex, age, disability and sexuality. It further stipulates that refugees should not be penalised for illegal entry or stay. This recognises that seeking asylum requires refugees to breach immigration rules. It specifically rules out arbitrary detention purely on the basis of seeking asylum. It provides 'that no one shall expel or return a refugee against his or her will, in any manner whatsoever, to a territory where he or she fears threats to life or freedom' (UNHCR Convention and Protocol Relating to the Status of Refugees).

Sex and gender are now included among grounds for persecution, and asylum law and the courts are bound to take into account the specificity of women's experiences. But women often have trouble convincing authorities that they deserve protection and their accounts of persecution are discredited by those who should grant them protection.

There are of course major reasons behind the movement of vast numbers of people from poor countries to developed nations, including impoverishment, climatic destruction and civil war and war lord violence. All contribute to what can only be called forced migration. Many have experienced violence directly – on themselves, their family and their community – and face dealing with fear for themselves and their children, loss of home and death of loved ones. Women may be fleeing sexual violence or forced prostitution as part of the religious or ethnic persecution they have suffered. The impression that the genuinely persecuted can be sorted out from among the refugees and clandestine immigrants looking for work, is erroneous. Whatever their experiences, great numbers of people are prepared to take enormous risks in leaving their country of origin; at time of writing their movement is sweeping through Europe.

To relieve pressure, ostensibly on social housing in London and areas around the ports, the National Asylum Support Service (NASS) was introduced in April 2000 as part of the Home Office, to replace the asylum teams from local authority social services departments. The change meant that resettlement policy was decided nationally with specific towns designated as places where new arrivals would be dispersed to specific cities across the UK, such as Handsworth and Smethwick, Kingston upon Hull and Stoke-on-Trent.

Social work in general involves exposure to the emotionally charged experiences of service users. In work with asylum seekers practitioners face not only their traumatic experiences but do so in a politicised context unlike any other area of social work practice (Robinson 2014: 1610). Robinson interviewed a number of practitioners working with voluntary organisations that shoulder much of the community-based work with asylum seekers and refugees. They described how difficult it was to maintain professional boundaries with service users who were so vulnerable. Their training had not prepared them for the human rights element in the work, including recording testimony of torture and trauma. At the same time they were trying to get people rehoused as quickly as possible, get their health assessed and organise other forms of support. Relationships with health and social care providers often meant confronting racist attitudes, ranging from dismissive comments to refusal of services. Working with those just released from detention, the lack of access to mainstream services and the rapid change in policies all made the work extremely stressful, made more so by the intensity of the work, high caseloads and poor supervision.

THE STRESS OF WORKING WITH REFUGEES

A social worker with asylum seekers said:

> And what's quite difficult is that a client is opening up, telling me everything, then the next client is opening up, telling me everything. And I can see up to 10 or 12 clients in a day and that can be . . . I mean I saw 50 . . . A couple of months ago I saw . . . in 8 days I saw 56 clients. And I was head wrecked.
>
> (from Robinson 2014: 1612)

Destitution among asylum seekers

For 'persons subject to immigration control', Section 115 of the Immigration and Asylum Act 1999 removes entitlement to means-tested benefits such as income support, income-based Job Seeker's Allowance, housing benefit and council tax benefit, as well as a range of family and disability benefits such as child benefit and disability living allowance. Importantly for social workers, provision of family support under Section 17 of the Children Act is not available to a dependent child and members of the child's asylum-seeking family where adequate accommodation or essential living needs are being provided under the Act's support system. From 2007, all new applicants have a named 'case owner' who is responsible for dealing with all aspects of their case from initial interview to final integration or removal. To bolster public confidence the application process is subject to tighter time-scales and more rigorous reporting of decisions taken at each stage.

Recent legislation has served to widen the gulf between the legal status of migrants and asylum seekers on the one hand and their rights to residence, work and benefits on the other. Conditions hedge eligibility to supports on every side as the concept of 'earned citizenship' has become more prominent, with permanent residence and access to full rights to work and welfare increasingly conditional on migrants showing economic self-sufficiency. These include new measures to limit EU nationals' right to benefits – a minimum earnings threshold, a 'genuine prospect of work test' and restrictions on entitlement to housing benefit, child benefit and Child Tax Credits for newly arrived EU 'jobseeker' nationals.

CASE STUDY: GEORGE

George is in his twenties. He arrived in Britain from his West African country of origin in 2006. Once he had made his claim for asylum in Liverpool, he was allocated National Asylum Support Service (NASS) housing in Manchester. When his initial claim for asylum was refused, several months after he first applied, his solicitor appealed. Waiting for the appeal to be heard he was able to stay in the same accommodation and his subsistence support continued. However the appeal was rejected, his support was terminated and he had to leave his NASS accommodation almost immediately. He was homeless and for more than two years was entirely dependent on friends to let him stay and to help him out with basic necessities.

The Immigration and Asylum Act 1999 and succeeding legislation can present social workers, social care managers and social care officers with some uncomfortable dilemmas. The system of immigration control is essentially underpinned by coercion of unwanted individuals, part of a total system that includes legal and economic surveillance by tying welfare provision to immigration status. Migrants are the one group in Britain that can be routinely detained indefinitely without charge or trial. In 2012, more than 28,000 individuals were held in immigration detention. Many were held for only a few days, but more than one-third were held for more than two months, and others had been detained for many months or years – the UK is one of the few European countries that puts no time limit on detention (Sands 2012).

Housing, education, social services and health services are all part of the control apparatus, compounded by social workers' general ignorance of immigration law (Hayes and Humphries 2004). Since providing services through the National Assistance Act 1948 or the NHS and Community Care Act 1990 is dependent on immigration status, this requires practitioners to investigate the immigration status of a person asking for a service, contrary to their professional code of ethics. There is also tension between asylum law and the Children Act 1989. That Act stipulates that the child's welfare is paramount in decisions affecting children, yet this principle does not automatically apply to children in immigration-linked cases. Nevertheless the Home Office, in making decisions regarding children of parents whose immigration status is in doubt, is obliged 'to consider' the matter of the child's welfare when deciding to expel children or parents. As Cohen (2001) reminds us, it is imperative for social workers to write welfare reports that address each of the points in the checklist of the child's welfare contained in the Children Act 1989 in cases of deportation.

Women asylum seekers

Refugees almost wholly come from countries where persecution, civil war, death threats, conflict and mass violence, both individual and communal, occur. Once in the UK they face an uphill task in rebuilding their lives because their access to resources is so constrained. This process is heavily gendered, based on different, gross assumptions about reasons for arrival. Women claiming asylum are expected to disclose their entire story, including any details about sexual violence, without any mistakes, on demand. They must do so to lawyers, Home Office staff and interpreters who may be men, and in environments including detention centres which are perceived as hostile and intimidating. For many vulnerable women this is extremely difficult. In one sample, many of the women had been persecuted by soldiers, police or prison guards in their country of origin, and had been raped and the victim of sexual violence, which carried shame and stigma in their home culture. Women in the Detained Fast Track have their case heard while they are in detention, often very soon after arrival in the UK, and may suffer post-traumatic stress syndrome, reliving earlier experiences of violence and imprisonment. If women are slow to disclose all the details of their persecution, or if they make mistakes in their accounts, they are often judged not to be credible, and will have their cases refused (Doyle 2014).

CASE STUDY: ELLA

Ella was forced into marriage at 19 to a distant relation of her father's who had no affection for her. In a country that had no laws against domestic violence she was regularly beaten by her husband – with the scars to prove it – but told to accept it as something women have to bear. She began to fear for her life and that of her 6-year-old daughter. She bought a plane ticket to Britain. On her first visit to the Croydon offices of the United Kingdom Border Agency (UKBA) she was told the officers didn't believe her and she was told to leave the building. She spent the night in a bus shelter, returning to the UKBA office at 4 am where she later completed her papers for a claim to asylum and was given directions to a hostel. On return to the UKBA offices ten days later, she was finger-printed, photographed and put into a van headed for a detention centre. Four days later, after another interview, her claim for asylum was refused. The grounds: because she did not know her husband's birthdate they deemed she was not actually married and therefore would not consider her evidence of abuse.

(adapted from Freud 2012)

REPORT ON CONTRACTS FOR ACCOMMODATION OF ASYLUM SEEKERS

In March 2012, the Department signed six new contracts for the provision of these services, collectively called COMPASS (Commercial and Operating Managers Procuring Asylum Support). It awarded G4S, Serco and Clearel contracts to supply accommodation services, with each awarded a contract to deliver these services in two of the six regions of the UK. The Department aimed to save around £140 million over seven years through the introduction of the new contractual arrangements; in 2012–13, it achieved a saving of £8 million. The new delivery model involves fewer and bigger housing providers than under the previous contracts.

* Only one of the three providers under COMPASS (Clearel) had any previous experience of the asylum housing sector. The contracts became fully operational in all areas by January 2013 following a transition period.

- G4S and Serco took on housing stock from previous suppliers of accommodation without carrying out inspections – and later found that many of the properties did not meet contractual quality standards.
- 20,000 asylum seekers were housed by the Department during the transition between the two contracted suppliers.
- Contractors were given inadequate information – take-up of asylum accommodation was higher than the Department predicted.
- Accommodated asylum seekers registered concerns about the quality of the accommodation where backlogs of maintenance and repairs were not addressed. The approach of some of the housing staff was also criticised for a poor understanding of users' needs.

(NAO COMPASS 2014: 6)

Unaccompanied child asylum seekers

Unaccompanied migrant children are those not only separated from their parents but not being cared for by an adult with legal or customary responsibility for doing so. While overall statistics are hard to come by for this group of children (numbers for example would include trafficked children and others separated by civil war), the number of unaccompanied children seeking asylum is recorded: in 2012 about 1,200 sought asylum; in 2015 the number had increased to 2,564. Around 2,150 unaccompanied migrant children were being cared for by local authorities (Joint Committee on Human Rights 2013). While few were granted formal refugee status, a large proportion were granted leave to remain on humanitarian grounds. In 2003, some 12,500 refugee children were deemed 'children in need' by local authorities – 6 per cent of all children in need. Of these some 2,400 were looked after by local authorities (Kohli 2007: 10–11). Of this number some 10 per cent were able to live independently with cash payments from local authority social service departments through Section 17 of the Children Act, while the others were fostered (70 per cent) or accommodated in children's homes or hostels (20 per cent; ibid.: 12).*

THE CHILD AS REFUGEE: UN CONVENTION ON THE RIGHTS OF THE CHILD (1989)

Article 221 of the UN Convention on the Rights of the Child (1989):

A child who is seeking refugee status or who is considered a refugee . . . shall, whether unaccompanied or accompanied by his or her parents or by another person, receive appropriate protection and humanitarian assistance . . . including help to trace the parents or other members of the family . . . in order to obtain information necessary for unification.

*In 2015–2016 the arrival of unaccompanied migrant children in great numbers from Syria raised the prospect of the compulsory dispersal of children across various local authorities, bringing extra work of settling disputes over age, the transport and relocation of children, and coordination with those authorities where the children first entered.

REFLECT AND DECIDE: SOCIAL WORK AND THE UNACCOMPANIED CHILD SEEKING ASYLUM

Bahri is 15 years old and is an unaccompanied refugee from Kosovo. His social worker gave him a travel card to go between his foster placement and his school – a journey involving a train and two buses. When his first foster placement broke down he had been offered a place at another school closer to where his new foster parents lived. This he declined and his school agreed that he should continue to attend there even though it acknowledged that he was unsettled in his behaviour. One day Bahri had a fight with a local boy who tore up his travel card. As a result Bahri had to walk home, which took him three hours. The next day he took a skewer to school and used it to threaten the boy who tore up his card. He was immediately suspended from school. Bahri said: 'He is the one who is to blame because he committed a terrible act on me [and] I was defending myself' (adapted from Kohli 2007: 140).

As Bahri's social worker what would the first tasks be? How would you talk to Bahri about the incident? Would you seek to move Bahri to another school? Would you seek to change the school's understanding of how to respond to Bahri? Would you bring in other resources or services to support or discipline Bahri?

Promoting inclusion with refugees and asylum seekers

The skills needed for effective work to reduce the exclusion experienced by refugees and asylum seekers are those needed in the other realms of this work: communication, assessment, building networks, resource finding, advocacy, mediation, support and counselling. The ecological model has clear implications for practice by getting the practitioner to focus on the relationship between the family and community, with school or early years centres as crucial institutional sources of support for children.

Kohli (2007) has conceptualised three domains for social work practice. While he has developed these in relation to unaccompanied children seeking asylum in Britain, they are useful in mapping the practice terrain for all refugees and asylum seekers.

The first is the *domain of cohesion* in which the primary focus is on the 'here and now', the practicalities of settlement such as providing shelter, care, food, money, schooling, medical support, welfare advice, a support network and ensuring good legal representation in relation to any claim for asylum. Social workers in this domain follow humanitarian efforts of non-governmental organisations (NGOs) abroad, offering material and practical help. Kohli describes them as 'realists, pragmatists' who want 'to deal with the present first, the future next and the past last' (Kohli 2007: 156).

The second is the *domain of connection* which focuses on resettlement of the 'inner world' of the refugee. Here social workers respond to the emotional distress of leaving the country of origin and help the person connect events, people and feelings that will assist in making sense of them. Kohli's observation of the young people he interviewed applies to many refugees and asylum seekers: while few needed psychiatric or therapeutic services, many were 'psychologically dishevelled as a consequence of dislocation and the shredding of roots' (ibid.: 156). The social work then is mindful of making connection between past and present and between inner and outer worlds, to free up emotions to cope with resettlement.

The third is the *domain of coherence* in which social workers frame the experiences of asylum seekers within a broader view of how children (and adults, we can add) cope with extraordinarily adverse circumstances by making the best use of their own strengths and capabilities. These workers – Kohli dubs them 'the Confederates' – look for and find resilience, express fondness and attachment towards them, making 'the line between friendship and professional help less distinct' and in so doing try to make the young person feel more at home (ibid.: 157).

Housing and community links

Housing is a key resource in the resettlement of asylum seekers and refugees. This is an area in which refugee community organisations may already be at work, particularly in London but also in the cities designated as dispersal areas, with social housing landlords and others setting up and managing accommodation schemes for refugees. These may start out by managing short-life property from local authorities. to which they then add systems of social support. The twin objectives of such schemes is to support tenancies and to help resettlement in the local community. In this, local colleges are vital – they provide access to training, education and employment. (In Stoke-on-Trent, for example, housing requests often focus on the area around the local college.) Placing people in safe areas is paramount. If settlement involves interim housing, then resettlement to permanent accommodation should be part of the broader plan. Some housing providers may be reluctant to take refugee tenants unless they know that there is a support package in place; any housing assistance should be tied to helping people negotiate their way around agencies.

GYPSIES AND TRAVELLERS

Gypsies and Irish Travellers,* who are among the most excluded minority ethnic groups, were for the first time officially recognised as an ethnic group in the 2011 UK census. In the wake of that census, statutory services included a 'Gypsy or Irish Traveller' category in their own ethnic monitoring procedures.

While it is difficult to quantify in any meaningful way the comparative degree to which specific groups are excluded, Gypsies and Travellers experience some of the most intense and compressed attributes of social exclusion. They suffer worse health, yet are less likely to receive effective health care. Life expectancy is 10–12 years below the national average and 18 per cent of Gypsy and Traveller mothers have experienced the death of a child, compared to less than 1 per cent of the general population. Forty-three per cent of children are eligible for free school meals in primary schools and 45 per cent in secondary schools. Twenty-two per cent of children have asthma compared to 5 per cent of the general population. Women live on average twelve years less than women in the general population and men ten years less.

*All the data in this and the following paragraphs are drawn from Cemlyn *et al.* 2009 and Allen 2012.

Twenty-five per cent of Gypsy and Traveller children are not enrolled in education and, for those that do attend, educational attainment is lower than for any other ethnic group and is still falling, particularly in secondary education where their participation is low and discrimination from school staff high. In 2011 just 12 per cent of Gypsy, Roma and Traveller pupils achieved five or more good GCSEs, including English and mathematics, compared with 58.2 per cent of all pupils. Children and young people also lack access to pre-school, out of school and leisure services. Research has noted accelerated criminalisation of young people, with disproportionate numbers of anti-social behaviour orders, and judicial perceptions about risk of absconding leading to remands in custody and secure accommodation.

As Cemlyn sums up traveller exclusion: 'There is an unquantified but substantial negative psychological impact on children who experience repeated brutal evictions, family tensions associated with insecure lifestyles and an unending stream of overt and extreme hostility from the wider population' (Cemlyn *et al.* 2009).

Travellers face barriers in accessing mainstream social services – difficulties with literacy and lack of digital contact inhibit getting information about services; and with children placed in care outside the family there is little attempt to shore up their Gypsy or Traveller identity. Social work intervention itself leans more toward control and less toward family support. There are also conflicts over norms. Conditionality in the welfare system embodies behavioural expectations in relation to parenting standards and child behaviour at variance with travelling family experiences. Children and young people engage in caring and economic responsibilities at a younger age in ways that are viewed by local authorities as potentially dangerous. Child safeguarding procedures, linked to a conception of adequate parenting and individual children's rights, fail to look ecologically at the evictions, harassment and dangers of temporary stopping places that travelling families face (ibid.)

Specialist teams need to bridge the inevitable conflicts and barriers by engaging Gypsy and travelling communities, building trust and exchanging information. The aim is to support cultural strengths in their own approaches to problem solving, and to promote the integration of child protection with family support. Family group conferences are one way to solve child protection issues within the family network.

Specialist teams can also aim at community-level work, bringing inequalities to light as well as adopting an educative and advocacy role on behalf of the community, for example in relation to malicious child protection referrals or local conflicts over camps on unauthorised sites. Cemlyn argues that the control elements of social work, particularly child protection, should not be handled directly by a specialist team but should retain trust-building, advocacy and educative roles. The obvious difficulty in this is that, when faced with a child who has suffered, or is likely to suffer, significant harm, the sudden transfer of the work to a safeguarding team, with little or none of the relational trust or community understanding, would entail the loss of faith in services that the specialist team had endeavoured to build up.

TRAVELLERS, ROMA AND GYPSY CHILDREN IN CARE

Relatively few Traveller and Gypsy children are taken into care – but among the travelling community the sense that it could happen is widespread. Travellers are aware that children services personnel frequently regard them as 'outside the outsiders' and hold fixed ideas about their lifestyle, child-rearing practices, and attitude toward school attendance.

> I remember as soon as they [my parents] were gone I was pushed into a bath and scrubbed because they told me I was dirty because I was from a Traveller family . . . I had beautifully thick, long black hair. If you stood me in a line with the other girls you could tell that I was a Traveller because of my hair. The care workers cut it all off because they said it was dirty.
>
> (adapted from Allen 2012: 91)

Personal prejudices of social workers and child-care staff play an outsize role, particularly the idea of rescuing children from an undeserved lifestyle. The child's wishes and freedom to choose can be overlooked.

CASE STUDY: HARINGEY TRAVELLING PEOPLE'S TEAM

The team's work embraces services for Traveller children and family joint casework, vulnerable adults casework, education support work, community group work, youth work and welfare rights work. On accommodation issues the team plays a key role in ensuring the cohesive and culturally appropriate management of the borough's Traveller sites, engagement with unauthorised encampments and Traveller housing support. The team also provides support for health issues, child poverty needs assessments and community engagement and input into service provision.

KEY POINTS

❑ Racism continues to play a powerful role in the social exclusion of ethnic minorities and the areas where they live; it finds new targets and new ways of expressing itself.

❑ The implications of institutional racism need to be addressed by service organisations, private, public and voluntary.

❑ The concept of community cohesion is at variance with the concept of institutional racism in that cultural and ethnic differences are seen as problems in so far as they disrupt the uniformity of citizenship. On the other hand it also focuses on segregation and seeks to build bridges between ethnic communities.

❏   The rights of refugees and asylum seekers, guaranteed under the UN Convention on Refugees, are often set aside in the process of claiming asylum. A rights-based practice in support of claimants is clearly indicated, particularly for women and unaccompanied children who have virtually no voice within the system.

❏   Gypsies and Irish Travellers have the lowest educational attainment and poorest health of any ethnic minority. Dedicated teams working with them are one promising practice solution.

KEY READING

Michael Lavelette and Laura Penketh, *Race, Racism and Social Work* (Policy Press, 2013). As a profession social work has been in the forefront of recognising racism and its own flawed response. This is the standard work by authors long in the field.

Kamena Dorling, Marchu Girma and Natasha Walter, *Refused: The Experiences of Women Denied Asylum in the UK* (Women for Refugee Women, 2012). Women asylum seekers – if one could actually measure this sort of thing – are among the most excluded groups in Britain. This report graphically spells out their plight and in doing so the plight of many asylum seekers. The implications for social work are numerous.

Ravi Kohli, *Social Work with Unaccompanied Asylum Seeking Children* (Palgrave Macmillan, 2007) is more relevant than ever – full of case studies and analysis as to what practitioners' response should be.

LEARNING IN PRACTICE

Tackling social exclusion is complex, with multiple targets for intervention set over sustained periods of time involving an array of partners including, prominently, service users. The work requires continuous learning – refitting itself not just with new skills but with new aspirations and new philosophies as to what it is trying to achieve long term. Evaluation offers an effective way to learn from practice; in fact the word 'learning' is partner to 'evaluating' as it better describes what the main purpose of evaluation should be – an educative process through which the practitioner, team and organisation are enabled to see clearly and without illusion the effects of their own work and the ways they can improve on that work.

Evaluating projects in open, dynamic systems such as those social work engages with is an uncertain activity facing several challenges. Projects change within an ever-changing environment. Baselines – the start point for measuring the progress of a particular project or action – are difficult to establish. Social work achieves what it does through developing rapport with users, helping them identify problems and assemble a narrative of their lives – all are difficult to measure with any sense of objectivity. In particular, social work evaluations have tended to concentrate on the *quality* of the service, as it is understood by practitioners, partners and stakeholders involved in delivery, rather than on *outcomes* – the impact of that service on the quality of life of users (Blom and Moren 2012).

BASIC EVALUATION TECHNIQUES

The distinctive purpose of evaluation is to improve practice. Much social work commentary on evaluation sees it as an extended form of critical reflection that focuses on the experience of interviewing, assessment and care planning. Qualitative studies are favoured, assembling opinions, reflections and views from practitioners and users along thematic lines. Qualitative methods – case studies, narratives, interviews, participant observation – create the 'extraordinary intimate acquaintance' between researcher and user (Shaw 2011: 93). They get stories told, views articulated, feelings elaborated in relation to the functional elements of casework.

Evaluating projects tackling exclusion is of a different order. While qualitative studies are important to gain insight on how users and workers regard a particular initiative, the aim must be to establish how observed outcomes are caused by, or in some way related to, the particular programme being evaluated. To do that, evaluators need to consider how those outcomes would have been different had the programme *not* been implemented. To establish this, many evaluations use 'before and after' estimates, defining 'baseline' or start-point data, then gathering fresh data after a programme has run for a period of time (Hollister 2007). The conclusion reached is whether outcomes have been met and within the time-frames specified.

Evaluators sometimes construct comparison groups – groups of individuals with characteristics similar to those who are participating in the programme – and then compare the outcomes for the two groups, those who had been part of the programme and those who had not (Hollister 2007). Sometimes specified outcomes are broken down further into specific 'indicators' that lend themselves more readily to quantification and tabulation. Many of the recent national evaluations of major government programmes, such as Sure Start local programmes, and Children's Fund, have used this basic approach.

OUTPUTS, INPUTS AND OUTCOMES: A HOT LUNCH PROGRAMME FOR OLDER PEOPLE

Outcomes encapsulate what a programme intends to achieve for service users, while *output* is what the service produces. For example, in the provision of twenty hot lunches served daily at a day centre for older people, the number of lunches is the output. The *inputs* are the resources devoted to delivering the lunches – staff hours, volunteer hours and the budget for food purchase and the like. The *outcome* is to improve the nutrition of those who attend.

The output – the lunch – does not guarantee the outcome, and the extent to which the outcome is achieved should be the focus of evaluation. This is not as simple as one might think. The outcome – improved levels of nutrition – can be measured for those who attend, but even if found to be the case, it may be the result of factors other than the hot meal. Evaluation then would have to consider what other factors, apart from the lunch, may have contributed to the outcome.

The importance of getting outcomes right

In his important and widely read study of multiple evaluations of social work education Carpenter argued that it is

> insufficient to evaluate training according to whether or not the student enjoyed the presentations and found them informative, or to assume that it is adequate to establish that students acquired particular skills, in communication, for example, without investigating whether or not they were able to transfer those skills to practice. Further, since the ultimate purpose is to benefit service users and/or carers, a comprehensive evaluation should ideally ask whether training has made any difference to their lives.
>
> (Carpenter 2011: 125)

A similar principle applies to all social work evaluations – gathering opinion on the success or otherwise of a project, whether it was enjoyed and what users thought they gained from it, is only part of the job. The more difficult task is to determine whether specified outcomes have actually been achieved in practice.

CASE STUDY: EVALUATING A SMOKING CESSATION CAMPAIGN FOR NEW PARENTS

To evaluate a smoking cessation programme aimed at parents with young children within a particular neighbourhood, the first step could be to establish the rates of smoking among parents with infants under 12 months before the programme is launched, and then to compare these rates with rates of smoking after the programme had been running for say a two-year period.

Parents may say they learned a lot from it – but of course that is insufficient as evidence. If it was found that a reduction in parent smoking had taken place it would still not necessarily mean that the programme itself was responsible for the reduction in smoking rates since this could have been caused by other factors. For example the increased general awareness among the public at large about how bad smoking is for health might have contributed to the reduction during the same time span, with the prohibition on smoking in pubs and restaurants particularly calling attention to the effects of secondary smoking.

Alternative methods of evaluation

The field of evaluation has widened considerably from this basic comparative approach and has become so diverse that no one method is deemed more reliable than others. There are many different forms – from single case studies and process (or 'logic') models, discussed below, to large-scale, whole-programme evaluations conducted over a period of time, such as that of Sure Start (NESS 2012) or social work practices (Manthorpe *et al.* 2014). Some are built on qualitative data – often semi-structured interviews coded according to themes – while others are quantitative, relying on statistical evidence. Experimental design following models of natural sciences experimentation is difficult to put into practice for the obvious reason that one cannot control the experimental conditions as one can in a research laboratory. In a sense, however, it remains the 'gold standard' and the most sophisticated evaluations of large national programmes attempt to introduce at least some quantitative evidence through testing or randomised control trials.

Because there are now many ways to approach evaluation, each with their own justification and rationale, it is important to think carefully which approach to choose and what would be the consequences of that choice. What will an evaluation tell about the practice? Will its methods reflect the diversity of a partnership? What will its effect be on the action itself (Julkunen 2011)?

Top-down or bottom-up evaluation?

Selecting a particular research method pre-determines who gets to participate and in what form. It also assumes that the method, in the hands of the expert evaluator, will produce a reliable and objective finding. Method-driven evaluations are top-down; they do not adequately address issues and interests of stakeholders and are difficult to reproduce in a real-world context (Chen n.d.). Critics sometimes refer to these as 'black box' evaluation, since how the method produces reliable findings is hidden from view.

In reaction to top-down forms of evaluation, approaches have become more bottom-up, participative, dialogue-based techniques where those doing the evaluation meet with both those staffing the programme being evaluated and users. Bottom-up evaluation aims for 'reflexivity' – organisational self-understanding that develops as it explores the consequences of its own actions in pursuit of specific missions. Evaluation is not a matter of bringing in an expert (or expert team); it involves communication and construction of knowledge by all participants in a social project.

EVALUATION: WHAT DO WE WANT TO KNOW?

Key questions behind any evaluation are: What do we want to know? What do we need to know? Who is going to join with us in our quest for this knowledge? How are we going to set about gaining this knowledge? The aim may be to establish public recognition of a programme – for example funders of a project will want to know whether the objectives of the project are being achieved and whether their money is being spent efficiently. Or the aim may be to get the opinions of those who receive the service as to whether it gives them what they want. Or the aim might be for the organisation itself – simply to learn to do better that which is being done in everyday practice.

EVALUATION AND CULTURE CHANGE

Evaluation with all its variation is a major learning tool for both practitioners and their organisations. It complements rather than replaces the accumulated practice wisdom and tacit knowledge that practitioners have built up through experience within a service organisation. There is every reason, then, to build evaluation in at the ground level. Waiting for top-down initiatives from inside or outside the organisation separates evaluative learning from the ground level. As Wilkinson and Applebee put it:

> Means will become ends. Process improvement will be detached from outcomes and the focus will go internal. The predominating interest will once again be on inputs and top-down indicators of success. In no time we will have an array of indications that purport to measure the effectiveness of partnerships but that are themselves quite disconnected from the real need for partnership on the ground.
>
> (Wilkinson and Applebee 1999: 15–16)

Building practice experience through small initiatives and informal partnerships, and accumulating knowledge through evaluation, is an essential step. Discussing impact and the lessons learned from implementing specific programmes or initiatives within team meetings, and assembling data and evaluative material to reflect on and be stimulated by what occurs in practice, sets up the 'continuous feedback loop' so prized by theorists of the learning organisation.

The process of continuous knowledge building is underpinned by a capacity to understand the continuous cycle of gathering evidence and evaluating that evidence. This is rarely a straightforward process, particularly in a field involving multiple resources, multiple partners and a long time-frame for delivery. It is all the more necessary, then,

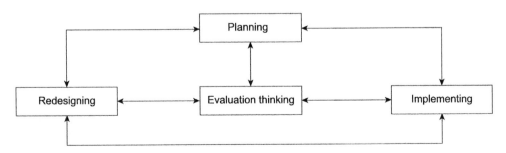

FIGURE 10.1   Evaluation: the key link in organisational learning (Frechtling 2007 reproduced with permission of John Wiley & Sons, Inc.)

for a learning organisation to be able to appraise different kinds of evidence, be able to understand how different factors influence decision making and how they impact what actually happens in the field.

Carpenter's review of a number of evaluations of social work education over two decades, drawn largely from the UK and the US, found that three-quarters of the studies only measured changes in attitudes and knowledge – as he put it, 'simple pre-post studies with one group of students' (Carpenter 2011: 125). The problems he found in social work education extend to the profession in the field, with the value of evaluations limited because observed outcomes cannot be ascribed exclusively to the intervention that is being evaluated (ibid.).

Sheldon and Chilvers (2001) make a number of suggestions that social work organisations can adopt for gathering evidence:

• Staff development systems, including supervision, should regularly draw on research to inform decisions about work with users or in projects. Questions should be regularly asked: 'so why are we proceeding in this way?' and 'on what evidence are you making this decision?'
• Make a range of support facilities available to assist staff in their efforts to keep abreast of relevant research in their field, with document supply facilities and summaries of evidence available.
• Practitioner attitudes need to include some personal responsibility for searching out and drawing on evidence of effectiveness.
• Develop collaborative arrangements between social service agencies and local universities and research institutes, so that each influences the work of the other, through joint seminars and work experience, and so that common purposes around social exclusion practice are understood and mutually interrogated.

Understanding complexity

Tackling social exclusion is complex and long-term – it is after all a product of the social and economic environment in which changes do not occur in linear fashion. Small changes in that environment, introduced by an initiative, may produce small changes, or very large changes, or no changes at all. It is all too easy to look at the social environment, for example of a disadvantaged neighbourhood, and break it down into a collection of factors – poor housing, anti-social behaviour, under-stimulated young children. So strong is our belief in analysis that we take these to make up the reality of that environment and lose sight of the total social system. But in this system outcomes are determined by multiple causes and these causes can combine in unpredictable ways, either reinforcing (for a large effect) or cancelling themselves out (for a negligible effect) (Byrne 1998).

The difference between *complicated* and *complex* is one reason why we find it difficult to understand how social interventions work. A task is complicated, because it involves a sequence of many different steps that are intricate and detailed. For example building an airliner requires following a pattern of rules, protocols and standards that must be scrupulously adhered to in order to ensure that the plane will fly safely. While they take some time to master, *once* these rules and standards are mastered, manufacturing the airliner can be done over and over again because the rules stay the same.

Complexity is not like that. It involves multiple potential outcomes, including those that are unforeseen, an ever-changing mix of resources and human inputs, and hidden relationships between circumstances and human agents. These are the conditions under which those who would struggle to reverse the many effects of long-standing social disadvantage, practice. A programme for young people who engage in anti-social behaviour will have multiple outcomes and other impacts not wholly predictable. In an initiative to promote the inclusion of a particular group of people within a social environment – for example young people congregating in a park every night – practitioners and local residents may be expecting a different set of outcomes – for example young people no longer meeting in visible groups – only to find that they have achieved others. The broader the objectives are, the wider the targets for intervention, the more complex and unpredictable the outcomes will be.

CASE STUDY: COMPLEXITY AND UNINTENDED CONSEQUENCES – WHEN DO BURGLARIES PEAK?

A community safety neighbourhood forum on a social housing estate reported that a number of youths were clustering on particular streets around 7pm in the evening. This seemed to coincide with an increase in burglaries in the area, according to residents, and the forum appealed for extra policing on the streets in the evenings and even called for dispersal orders to be issued. It was only some time later that a record was kept of when burglaries were happening and not just where. Examining the record after two months, the forum found that the peak time for burglaries was around 3.30 to 4 pm – just after school finished – and concentrating police activity in the evening inadvertently contributed to that.

EVALUATING SOCIAL EXCLUSION PROGRAMMES

As with any evaluation, there are difficulties in trying to evaluate the kinds of programmes that tackling social exclusion requires. First, as noted above, initiatives are complex, with large social objectives – bringing about social change – that call for a range of actions and resources. The effects of such initiatives are often difficult to track. How can you identify which input, resource or activity is responsible for any given outcome? Second, there are many different stakeholders in the form of service agencies' managers and practitioners, local politicians, a range of local organisations and their leaders, and residents with different interests and commitments. How do they arrive at agreed standards for evaluation? Third, initiatives take place over a much longer time-frame than the usual techniques are accustomed to handling. How can you link with certainty the outcomes in year four of an initiative to resources put in place in year one? There is presumably some relationship but of course other unplanned factors may have influenced outcomes three years later.

Tackling social exclusion draws on large-scale public efforts intended to be participative in process while at the same time committed to producing specific results. These efforts require the support of a wide range of stakeholders, all of whom need to be kept informed of progress toward outcomes and to have evidence that their involvement

– whether of time and energy or funding – is worthwhile. Neighbourhood residents in particular need to know whether the promises and hopes extended by particular initiatives are bearing fruit.

Several factors can make evaluation of social exclusion programmes a contested, protracted process. With multiple stakeholders conflicts of interest are bound to emerge. Evidence may be used selectively, deployed for particular purposes and not others. Politicians or local officials will want quick and visible wins, evaluators and researchers will be looking to augment their research profiles, while agencies will be prone to cherry-pick from the evidence base that best suits their service and defends their turf. Add to this mix the limits of evaluation 'science' and you have, in the words of Coote and colleagues: 'not the component parts of a single jigsaw . . . but bits from many different puzzles, most of which are incomplete' (Coote *et al.* 2004: 47). Whether evaluation is cast in the form of technical assistance or within a broader flow of knowledge building, some appraisal of a project through a transparent, trusted and widely understood process, where conflicting interests and competing philosophies are openly acknowledged, is essential (Hughes and Traynor 2000; Kubisch and Stone 2001).

Rossi *et al.* (2003) assert that evaluation 'is the systematic application of social research procedures for assessing the conceptualisation, design, implementation and utility of social intervention programmes'. Despite the confident ring in this definition, as we have already observed, there is no one way to evaluate a programme or initiative. All approaches have limitations. Just as it is quite possible to have unrealistically high expectations of what a programme can achieve, so it is unrealistic to expect that an evaluation will be able to assess definitively how well a programme has worked and why. Organisational learning is a two-way street: it requires evidence that is capable of generating learning as well as the organisational and practitioner capacity to learn from that evidence (Coote *et al.* 2004: 30).

Coote and her colleagues have summarised some of the perplexities that can beset practitioners in learning from evidence. One is the difficulty in weighing up the relative merits of different sources and types of knowledge. For example when is practice experience and tacit knowledge – the kind of knowledge picked up through experience that cannot be written down or even verbalised in formal propositions – a more reliable basis for judgement than published research findings or the opinion of an external evaluator? Another difficulty is the usefulness of the format that much evidence takes – abstract and removed from the day-to-day demands confronting practitioners.

Practitioners tend to give priority to delivering the practical outputs required by a programme and attempt to meet targets and other performance indicators rather than to reflect on longer-term broader outcomes and academic research (Coote *et al.* 2004: 33). In numerous interviews Coote and her colleagues found that practitioners needed more guidance on how to use evaluations and evidence and greater consistency across programmes in their approaches to evaluations. Evaluations need to be geared more closely to practice needs, with researchers focusing on questions that practitioners need answering rather than, as all too often, practitioners having to comb published evaluations for anything that might be relevant to their work (Coote *et al.* 2004: 35).

One can see the potential for conflicting views and interests in the most basic evaluative effort. Nevertheless any evaluation, including self-evaluation, should undertake four basic functions:

- Audit: did the programme do what it set out to achieve within budget?
- What was the level of satisfaction with the results – such as specific outputs and outcomes?
- Value for money – did the programme have an impact, did it make a difference in changing the set of social conditions it was targeting? Can it be clearly established that the programme was responsible for the changes effected?
- What were the elements of 'best practice' within the programme? Can comparisons be made with programmes elsewhere – or with what would have happened had no programme been introduced in the first place?

REFLECT AND DECIDE: EVALUATING A DOMESTIC VIOLENCE PROGRAMME

Police in a particular locality have begun a new initiative to counteract domestic violence, essentially based on arresting men who have committed violence on their partners for a second time – even when the incident is relatively minor. Discretion is removed from the individual police officer and/or social worker who are involved in the incident. In every incident the alleged perpetrator is arrested though they may not necessarily subsequently be charged.

The task is to develop some testable propositions regarding this initiative. Consider variations in community setting, family composition, sub-cultures, and economic and employment circumstances. Think also about gender difference and how it might impact both men and women encountering this programme. How might reactions vary in differing contexts? How might behaviour patterns then differ? Compare your thoughts with those of others given the same task.

(adapted from Tilley 2000)

Approaches to evaluation: logic models

There are many approaches to evaluating the effectiveness of complex programmes. They differ in intent: is the purpose of an evaluation truly objective or is it a tool for advocacy? Or in technique: is it to be qualitative or quantitative? Or in design: is it to be participatory, drawing on users' views, or quasi-experimental? Necessarily, then, a broad pragmatism is involved in choosing approaches to evaluation and key decisions need to be made at the outset about what information is to be gathered and how that information is to be assessed and interpreted. Moreover evaluation is more than simply answering the question whether a programme worked or not (a summative evaluation) – it should also inform improvement or modification as the project is unfolding (Frechtling 2007).

Logic models work through these questions as part of the evaluation process. Essentially they are a systematic and visual way of uncovering the relationships between the resources of a programme, the activities that the programme intends to carry out, and the changes or results it expects to achieve (Hollister 2007). The most basic logic model constructs a picture of how a programme is supposed to work. It uses words or

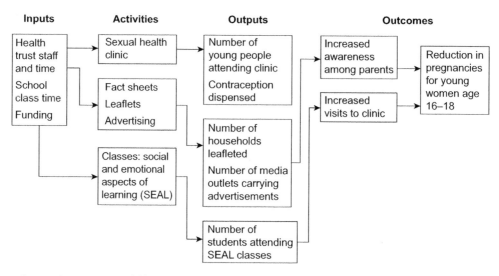

FIGURE 10.2 Logic model for a programme reducing pregnancies in young women, 16–18 (author)

pictures or both to describe the sequence of activities thought to bring about change and how these activities are linked to the results the programme is expected to achieve. It links the assumptions or 'theory' as to why a given programme will work to the actions that the programme will take based on this theory, and the expected short- and long-term outcomes that should be the result. Linking these elements causally helps an organisation identify all the steps it must take and how those steps lead to measurable outputs as well as less tangible outcomes.

REFLECT AND DECIDE: DESIGN AN EVALUATION

Design an evaluation of a scheme to place care leavers in 'suitable' accommodation (see Chapter 5). Specify outcomes for the care leavers that the scheme will achieve, i.e. what should the scheme deliver in terms of the wellbeing of those care leavers involved in it? Decide on the resources needed to meet those outcomes. Develop a 'theory of change' for the programme – why is the programme going to deliver these outcomes? Determine how the evaluation will know when the specific outcomes of the scheme have been achieved (or not).

Achieving Better Community Development

The ABCD model – Achieving Better Community Development – offers a simplified logic model. Within this approach Barr and Hashagen (2000) have incorporated many of the techniques required for evaluating projects with multiple outcomes achieved over time and an important role for services in achieving them.

The ABCD model works, as any logic model does, on four variables: inputs, processes, outputs and outcomes. Inputs are the range of resources and tools that are available from within the community or brought in by outside agencies working in support of community development. Such resources move well beyond funding to include:

- people's time, motivation and energy
- skills, knowledge and understanding
- trust within the neighbourhood
- networks
- leadership.

Stakeholders from outside the community bring resources such as a policy framework, expertise and training, additional funding and coordination. Processes are defined as those actions that need to take place to direct inputs towards specified outcomes. In this framework the central process is one of 'community empowerment', which embraces four components: personal development for individuals, 'positive action' for social justice and social inclusion, community organisation and the effectiveness of community-based groups, and gaining power and influence at local level. This empowerment process can be seen as the way in which inputs are used to develop the ability of the community to achieve change (Barr and Hashagen 2000: 61).

Outputs are the product of community empowerment, the specific actions that relate to economic, social, environmental or political issues of the locality. These outputs may include social service development, a safe and healthy community, or increased citizen control over services and political developments.

Outcomes are the consequences of the outputs relating to the improvement in the quality of life of the locality. Evaluation poses critical questions for each stage. What are the inputs to community development activity, and how do they change with the progress of action? How well are the inputs applied to the process of community empowerment? What are the outputs and outcomes? How is empowerment used to influence the quality of community life? (ibid.: 62).

To answer such questions some notion of a starting point or baseline has to be established as well as a number of indicators that will provide yardsticks as to what is being achieved. Once a baseline has been established, the evaluation task then requires

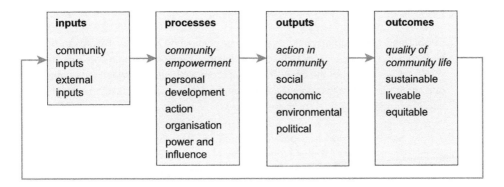

FIGURE 10.3   ABCD model of evaluation (Barr and Hashagen 2000)

information to be gathered and assessed. Gathering information is the crucial stage, requiring advance planning. You need to know what type of information is required, for example whether facts or opinion, and who you want to obtain information from, for example from users, local residents or community representatives. Information can be obtained by:

- Observation, that is, having an observer present when key events occur either as a participant-observer or as a non-participant.
- Asking questions – through questionnaires, face-to-face interviews, consultations or focus groups. Barr and Hashagen have sound advice as to how to gather information for evaluation:

  - be focused by asking relevant questions about specific activities
  - keep it as simple as possible
  - look for emerging themes by interpreting findings
  - offer choices and options to those you are seeking information from, such as ranking the importance of items
  - use innovative techniques such as tapes, photographs, exhibitions, physical representations, diagrams or storytelling.

(Barr and Hashogen 2000)

REFLECT AND DECIDE: EVALUATING A COMMUNITY RESOURCE CENTRE

A community resource centre on a low-income housing estate in east London is housed in a one-storey brick building, built around 1960. It is owned by the local authority but has been leased for a small sum to a consortium of agencies and local residents who have ambitious plans for it. The consortium has worked out a number of objectives that it thinks will provide what local people want from such a centre; it also reflects much of the new thinking around 'neighbourhood renewal'. One set of objectives is to increase the 'social strengths' of the estate by:

- Enabling residents to participate fully in the decision making and delivery of local services.
- Establishing sustainable structures to deliver community services. It wants to do this by increasing community capacity and facilities so that local people can take 'ownership' and leadership of the area, improving communication between the community and service providers to create more responsive services and to develop a neighbourhood management model for those services.

The only member of staff is a part-time caretaker. The resource centre is well used although the activities that take place there do not always seem to further the consortium's objectives. Among the activities that take place within it are the following:

- a luncheon club for older citizens four days a week
- occasional cultural activities for the substantial local Bengali population in the evening
- an after-school club for children up to the age of 14
- a training course in IT skills for women
- a youth club two nights a week
- a venue for local community groups to meet.

Plan a brief evaluation of the centre. Who do you think would be among the principal stakeholders and involved in the evaluation? What and who are the inputs? As far as the set of objectives is concerned, what indicators would you look for to measure any progress? What kind of information or data would you need and how would you go about collecting it? How would you present this information to users of the centre and to members of the consortium itself to make it a useful learning tool?

Theory of change and theory-driven evaluation

Theory of change is an approach to evaluation that shares many elements of a logic model. It acknowledges the complexity of a multi-pronged, multi-agency programme by pinpointing the specific interventions of a given programme and how they are intended to deliver the long-term outcomes. Essentially the theory of change approach asks certain questions of all participants in a project that tackles exclusion:

- Why is this project going to work?
- What are the theories that will make the project effective and achieve the (often complicated) social objectives that the project aspires to over the time span?
- How will you be able to show the outside world that the project has succeeded?

The phrase 'theory of change' means simply making clear and bringing into the open those theories on which the initiative is basing its plans: what are the concepts behind the programme that will ensure that the various outcomes identified will be reached over the period of time projected? Theory of change evaluation, in common with logic models, asks that projects first establish long-term outcomes and work backwards from these so that intermediate and then early outcomes relate to those long-term objectives. In terms of theorising why a planned programme should work, there are four potential sources of theory: (i) theories already established through research; (ii) implicit or practice theories developed by those close to the programme; (iii) theories drawn from observations of a programme already in operation; and (iv) exploratory research to test critical assumptions that underpin a particular theory.

There are three virtues in the theory of change approach. First the evaluator works from the beginning jointly with all stakeholders – local residents, practitioners, managers, councillors – as they shape up the long-term outcomes of any initiative. Second, in doing this the evaluator helps make explicit what theories are being drawn on to allow stakeholders to have confidence that those outcomes will be reached. Third, the theory of change can blend both process and hard outcomes in framing the first step, that is to say the long-term objectives (Hughes and Traynor 2000). On the other hand critics have said that it can be cumbersome in practice because it strives to factor in all the different stakeholders' points of view as well as the full array of inputs and resources. As an evaluative process, then, it can take a great deal of time and require skilled facilitation if the theory of change is to work (Coote *et al.* 2004).

TWO KEY QUESTIONS POSED BY THEORY-DRIVEN EVALUATION

1   The why question: why does the intervention affect the outcomes? In other words why will the particular programme succeed in overcoming the problem?
2   The how question: how are the contextual factors and programme activities organised so that the programme can be implemented?

Programme theory should be plausible (i.e. having the outward appearance of truth, reason, or credibility) and stipulate the cause-and-effect sequence through which actions are presumed to produce long-term outcomes or benefits. Theory-driven models are intended to integrate systems thinking in developing programme theory, taking into account contextual and other factors ostensibly external to the programme but that may influence its effectiveness (Coryn *et al.* 2011).

Critics of theory-driven evaluation are sceptical that such theories can be articulated, arguing (a) it is not really possible and (b) they are not needed in any case. What matters, they say, is whether a programme is effective – does what it sets out to do. They cite aspirin as an example – no one really knows why it achieves improvement to a range of health outcomes but it is well established that it does.

REFLECT AND DECIDE: SOCIAL WORK PRACTICES

Social work practices were an innovation first suggested in 2007. They rested on the theory that smaller social worker-led organisations, independent of local authorities, would (i) improve the morale and retention of children's social workers; (ii) reduce bureaucracy; and (iii) facilitate professional decision making. The theories in short had to do with improving the practitioners' work environment. It was hypothesised that these three effects would have a positive impact on outcomes for children and young people.

On the basis of this theorising five pilot social work practices were set up in 2010. Not long after, they were then extended to social care work – with similar reasoning: they would allow practitioners to spend more time with individuals, take decisions closer to users thereby making the service more responsive, reduce bureaucratic burden on individual social workers, and provide financial flexibility allowing workers to think creatively about resource use.

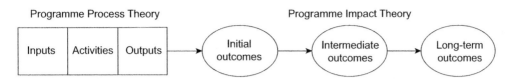

FIGURE 10.4a   Linear programme theory (Coryn *et al.* 2011; reproduced under the terms of the STM Permissions Guidelines)

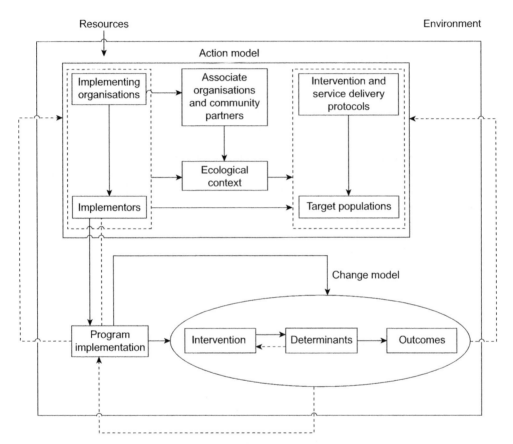

FIGURE 10.4b   Context-aware programme theory (Coryn *et al.* 2011; reproduced under the terms of the STM Permissions Guidelines)

Realist evaluation

Programmes tackling social exclusion are embedded in social systems and it is through the workings of systems of social relationships that changes in behaviours, events and social conditions are effected. Realist evaluation encompasses the systems and context within which programmes are embedded by addressing the issues of 'for whom' and 'in what circumstances' a programme will work. Some contexts will be supportive to the programme theory and some will not. This gives realist evaluation the crucial task of sorting the one kind of context from the other. It asks the question: given a specific context is the basic plan sound, plausible, durable, practical and, above all, valid?

Realist evaluation assumes that programmes cannot be isolated from their context over time. Externalities get in the way – unanticipated events, political change, personnel moves, media coverage, technological change, and performance management innovations all require programmes to be adaptable to the ever-changing environment. No two programmes are ever implemented in the same way. Nor is realist evaluation preoccupied with the question of whether programmes 'work'. Programmes *per se* do not work – it is the resources they provide that make them work. How those involved in a programme perceive and carry out the strategy is a central feature of realist research (Pawson and Tilley 1997).

Logic models, theory of change models and realist evaluation (Pawson and Tilley 1997) share a great deal in common, starting with the realisation that there is no 'black box' which can deliver a reliable objective set of findings regarding a complex social programme. All three approaches involve holistic assessment – taking into account contextual factors as well as causal relationships between actions taken under the programme and outcomes achieved. Their start point is with the theory behind the programme, identifying stakeholders' implicit and explicit assumptions on what actions are required to solve a problem and why the problem will respond to those actions (Chen 2005). The evaluation strategy is to assist stakeholders in clarifying the mechanisms and the contextual factors essential to their programme's success. They probe strengths and weaknesses of assumptions as to cause and effect – 'if we do this then that should happen' – and in so doing clarify for participating partners how the programme is supposed to work and what adjustments need to be made to make it more effective. The difference between a basic, linear evaluation and a 'context rich' evaluation can be seen in Figures 10.4a and 10.4b.

The practitioner as change agent in the learning organisation

It is tempting to think that practitioners can wait until someone fires the 'time to start tackling social exclusion' gun before taking forward elements of the practice outlined in this book. But that is not a luxury they have. The practitioner role should be one of catalyst and change agent regardless of position in the organisation. But to do this, an understanding of the 'self in the sea of change', to use Gerald Smale's phrase, is needed, to work with the changes in approach and vision, large and small, that tackling social exclusion requires. Smale frames three important questions that need answers:

1   Are the people you work with active or passive? Will they enthusiastically join, and perhaps lead, innovation or will they resist and have change imposed upon them? Smale reminds us that 'to have the rug pulled out from under you is a very different experience from coming to a decision to reject the old flooring and choose a new carpet' (Smale 1998: 122). In other words imposed or coerced change generates opposition and takes a lot of time to get over.

2   Does the innovation produce a change of identity? The degree of change determines the amount of learning and unlearning that staff will have to do. Tasks

will be upgraded and downgraded. Retaining autonomy, respect, dignity in the organisation and breadth of responsibility are all critical factors – often as important as remuneration in a period of change.

3   What do key people win or lose? To understand the impact of change on colleagues and others you work with, for example from other agencies in a prospective partnership, ask who is experiencing what aspect of change as a 'gain' or a 'loss'? What can you do to help people recognise real gains and build commitment to the new solutions and new situations?

Tackling social exclusion does mean at times going outside the grain of current practice – tying practice more closely to social justice and moral understanding of fairness, thinking hard about what constitutes 'preventive work' as opposed to 'defensive work', focusing more on collective and neighbourhood-level responses to social problems. Yet it is worth remembering that even in large social service organisations there is no 'single author' writing the script for what the organisation is to do and that the single social worker, the manager, the team, have more authority, power and influence than might be imagined.

Moreover the direction of any organisation is more open to change than one might think, with choices continually before it as to whether to follow one direction or another. It is open to practitioners always to create alternative networks, to find out who in the organisation is of like mind that one can speak to, and to decide on what information to give to that person. Watching out for how the whole enterprise of reducing social exclusion in Britain all joins up – even when doing just the small corner of it that comes a practitioner's way as they follow their day-to-day roles and tasks – means they should be ready to supply the message to whoever will listen.

KEY POINTS

❑   Evaluation in its broadest sense is about practice learning.

❑   Initiatives to tackle social exclusion are complex, bringing different kinds of intervention together. This makes evaluation also complex.

❑   There are differences in types of evaluation: top-down, based on expertise and management-stipulated requirements, and participative, bottom-up methods which are negotiated with all stakeholders including users. Both are needed – the objective is learning but also to gather hard evidence as to whether a specific programme is producing the outcomes desired.

❑   Specifying outcomes for a programme is critical, as is developing an underlying explanation (or 'theory') as to why the programme will achieve them.

❑   Logic models, including Achieving Better Community Development, theory of change models and realist models of evaluation are all receptive to wide participation. They also require thinking as to the underlying explanation of why a programme will work, while being sensitive to changing environment and context.

KEY READING

Ray Pawson and Nick Tilley, *Realistic Evaluation* (Sage, 1997).
Ian Shaw, *Evaluating in Practice* (Ashgate, 2011).
Missing thus far from both the practitioner and scholarly social work literature are robust schemes for evaluating the ecological approach.

BIBLIOGRAPHY

Acheson, D. (1998) *Independent Inquiry into Inequalities in Health*. London: The Stationery Office.

Age UK (2012) *Loneliness – the State We're in*. Oxfordshire: Age UK.

Age UK (2014) *Care in Crisis 2014*, www.ageuk.org.uk/Documents/EN-GB/Campaigns/CIC/Care_in_Crisis_report_2014.pdf?epslanguage=en-GB?dtrk%3Dtrue (accessed 3 March 2015).

Age UK (n.d.) *Loneliness and Isolation: Evidence review*, www.ageuk.org.uk/documents/en-gb/for-professionals/evidence_review_loneliness_and_isolation.pdf?dtrk=true (accessed 2 December 2014).

Alexander, A. (2000) *Mentoring Schemes for Young People – Handbook*. Brighton and London: Pavilion and National Children's Bureau.

Alinsky, S. (1971; revised 1989) *Rules for Radicals: A pragmatic primer for realistic radicals*. New York: Vintage Books.

Allen, D. (2012) Gypsies and Travellers and social policy: marginality and insignificance. A case study of Gypsy and Traveller children in care. In Richardson, J. and Ryder, A. (eds) *Gypsies and Travellers: Empowerment and inclusion in British society*. Bristol: Policy Press.

Allen, G. (2011) *Early Intervention: The next steps*. London: Department for Work and Pensions.

Ames, A., Powell, H., Crouch J. and Tse, D. (2007) *Anti-Social Behaviour: People, place and perceptions*. London: IPSOS Mori.

Anastacio, J., Gidley, B., Hart, L., Keith, M., Mayom, M. and Kowarzik, U. (2000) *Reflecting Realities: Participants' perspectives on integrated communities and sustainable development*. Bristol: Policy Press.

Anonymous (2011) *Nursing Standard* 25, 45, 8.

Arnstein, S. (1969) A ladder of citizen participation. *Journal of the American Institute of Planners* 35, 4, 216–224.

Atkinson, A., Cantillon, B., Marlier, E. and Nolan, B. (2002) *Social Indicators: The EU and social inclusion*. Oxford: Oxford University Press.

Atkinson, M., Jones, M. and Lamont, E. (2007) *Multi-agency Working and its Implications for Practice: A review of the literature*. Reading: CfBT Education Trust (NFER).

Axford, N. (2010) Is social exclusion a useful concept in children's services? *British Journal of Social Work* 40, 3, 737–754.

Axford, N., Lehtonen, M., Kaoukjo, D., Tobin, K. and Berry, V. (2012) Engaging parents in parenting programs: Lessons from research and practice. *Children and Youth Services Review* 34, 10, 2061–2071.

Ball, S. and Vincent, C. (1998) 'I heard it on the grapevine': 'hot' knowledge and school choice. *British Journal of Sociology of Education* 19, 3, 377–400.

Barnardo's (2014a) *On My Own: The accommodation needs of young people leaving care in England*. London: Barnardo's.

Barnardo's (2014b) *Hidden in Plain Sight: Research on the sexual exploitation of boys and young men: A UK scoping study*. London: Barnardo's.

Barnes, J. (2007) *Down Our Way: The relevance of neighbourhoods for parenting and child development*. Chichester: Wiley.

Barnes, J., Katz, I., Korbin, J. and O'Brien, M. (2006) *Children and Families in Communities: Theory, research, policy and practice*. Chichester: Wiley.

Barr, A. and Hashagen, S. (2000) *Achieving Better Community Development: Trainer's resource pack*. London: Community Development Foundation Publications.

Barr, A., Drysdale, J. and Henderson, P. (1997) *Towards Caring Communities: Community development and community care*. Brighton: Pavilion.

Barr, A., Stenhouse, C. and Henderson, P. (2001) *Caring Communities: A challenge for social inclusion*. York: Joseph Rowntree Foundation.

BASE (2014) The Use of Personal Budgets for Employment Support (NDTi), http://base-uk.org/sites/base-uk.org/files/knowledge/Personal%20Budgets%20and%20Supported%20Employment/pbs_and_employment_research_report_v2_4th_june_2014.pdf).

Bateman, N. (2005) *Practising Welfare Rights*. Abingdon: Routledge.

Beck, U. and Beck-Gernsheim, E. (2002) *Individualisation: Institutionalized individualism and its social and political consequences*. London: Sage.

Beckett, H., with Brodie, I., Factor, F., Melrose, M., Pearce, J., Pitts, J., Shuker, L. and Warrington, C. (2013) 'It's wrong . . . but you get used to it'. Bedford: Children's Commissioner and University of Bedfordshire.

Bennett, K., Beynon, H. and Hudson, R. (2000) *Coalfields Regeneration: Dealing with the consequences of industrial decline*. Bristol: Joseph Rowntree Foundation and the Policy Press.

Berelowitz, S., Clifton, J., Firimin, C., Gulyurtlu, S. and Edwards, G. (2013) *'If Only Someone Had Listened': Inquiry into child sexual exploitation in gangs and groups*. London: Children's Commissioner.

Beresford, P. (2012) The theory and philosophy behind user involvement. In Beresford, P. and Carr, S. (eds) *Social Care, Service Users and User Involvement*. London: Jessica Kingsley Publishers.

Berger, L., Font, S., Slack, K. and Waldfogel, J. (2013) *Income and Child Maltreatment: Evidence from the Earned Income Tax Credit*. Presentation at the Annual Meeting of the Association of Public Policy Analysis and Management.

Berger, L., Paxson, C. and Waldfogel, J. (2009) Mothers, men and child protective services involvement. *Child Maltreatment* 14, 263–276.

Biestek, F. (1961) *The Casework Relationship*. London: Allen & Unwin.

Bird, K. and Simkin, A. (2014) *Guide to Service User and Carer Involvement in Social Care Commissioning*. Exeter: Devon County Council.

Blackburn, C., Spencer, N. and Read, J. (2010) Prevalence of childhood disability and the characteristics and circumstances of disabled children in the UK: Secondary analysis of the Family Resources Survey. *BMC Pediatrics* 10, 21.

Blau, P. (1960) Structural effects. *American Sociological Review* 25, 2, 178–193.

Blom, B. and Moren, S. (2012) The evaluation of quality in social work practice. *Nordic Journal of Social Research* 3, 71–87.

Blomberg, H., Kroll, C., Kallio, J. and Erola, J. (2013) Social workers' perceptions of the causes of poverty in the Nordic countries. *Journal of European Social Policy* 23, 1, 68–82.

Blood, I. (2013) *A Better Life: Valuing our later years*. York: Joseph Rowntree Foundation.

Blood, I., Pannell, J. and Copeman, I. (2012) *Whose responsibility? Boundaries of roles and responsibilities in housing with care*. York: Joseph Rowntree Foundation.

Blow, C. (2014) Poverty is not a state of mind. *New York Times*, 18 May.

Blow, C. (2015) Confederate flags and institutional racism. *New York Times*, 24 June.

Blyth, M. (2014) *Austerity: The history of a dangerous idea*. Oxford: Oxford University Press.

Bowers, H. (2013) *Widening Choices for Older People with High Support Needs*. York: Joseph Rowntree Foundation.

Boyle, G. (2014) Recognising the agency of people with dementia. *Disability and Society* 29, 7, 1130–1144.

Bradshaw, J. (2015) Child poverty and well-being. Liverpool Children's Summit, 19 March.

Bradshaw, J. and Main, G. (2014) Austerity: Children are the victims in the UK. Paper presented at the Social Policy Association Annual Conference, University of Sheffield, 15 July.

Bradshaw, J. and Richardson, D. (2009) An index of child well-being in Europe. *Child Indicators Research* 2, 3, 319–351.

Brandon, M., Bailey, S., Belderson, P., Gardiner, R., Sidebotham, P., Dodsworth, J., Warren, C. and Back, J. (2009) *Understanding Serious Case Reviews and Their Impact*. London: Department for Children, Schools and Families.

Brandon, M., Sidebotham, P., Bailey, S., Belderson, P., Hawley, C., Ellis, C. and Megson, M. (2012) *New Learning from Serious Case Reviews: A two-year report for 2009–2011*. London: Department for Education Research Brief.

Braye, S. and Preston-Shoot, M. (1995) *Empowering Practice in Social Care*. London: Jessica Kingsley Publishers.

Brewer, M., Browne, J. and Joyce, R. (2011) *Child and Working-Age Poverty from 2010 to 2020*. London: Institute of Fiscal Studies.

Briggs, S. and Hingley-Jones, H. (2013) Reconsidering adolescent subjectivity: A 'practice-near' approach to the study of adolescents, including those with severe learning disabilities. *British Journal of Social Work* 43, 64–80.

Briggs, X. (1997) Social capital and the cities: Advice to change agents. International Workshop on Community Building, Bellagio, Italy.

—— (2002) *The Will and the Way: Local partnerships, political strategy and the well-being of America's children and youth*. Cambridge, MA: Harvard University Faculty Resource Working Papers.

—— (2004) *Desegregating the City: Issues, strategies and blind spots in comparative perspective*. Cape Town: Isandla Institute.

British Association of Social Workers (2012) *The Code of Ethics for Social Work Values and Ethical Principles*, http://cdn.basw.co.uk/upload/basw_112315-7.pdf (accessed 20 January 2014).

Brodie, E. and others (2011) *Pathways through Participation: What creates and sustains active citizenship?* London: NCVO and Institute for Volunteering Research.

Bronfenbrenner, U. (1979) *The Ecology of Human Development*. Cambridge, MA: Harvard University Press.

Brooks-Gunn, I., Duncan, G. and Aber, L. (eds) (1997) *Neighborhood Poverty: Context and consequences for children*. New York: Russell Sage Foundation.

Brooks-Gunn, J., Schneider, W. and Waldfogel, J. (2013) The effect of the great recession on the risk of child maltreatment. *Child Abuse and Neglect* 37, 10, 721–729.

Browne, K., Bakshi, L. and Lim, J. (2012) There's no point in doing research if no one wants to listen: Identifying LGBT needs and effecting positive social change for LGBT people in Brighton and Hove. In Beresford, P. and Carr, S. (eds) *Service Users and User Involvement*. London: Jessica Kingsley Publishers.

Browning, C. and Cagney, K. (2002) Neighborhood structural disadvantage, collective efficacy, and self-rated physical health in an urban setting. *Journal of Health and Social Behaviour* 43, 388–399.

Bullock, H. (2004) From the front lines of welfare reform: An analysis of social worker and welfare recipient attitudes. *Journal of Social Psychology* 144, 6, 571–588.

Bunting, M. (2006) It takes more than tea and biscuits to overcome indifference and fear. *Guardian*, 16 November.

Burchardt, T., Le Grand, J. and Piachaud, D. (1999) Social exclusion in Britain 1991–1995. *Social Policy and Administration* 33, 3, 227–244.

—— (2002) Degrees of exclusion: Developing a dynamic, multidimensional measure. In Hills, J., LeGrand, J. and Piachaud, D. (eds) *Understanding Social Exclusion*. Oxford: Oxford University Press.

Burchardt, T., Obolesckaya, P. and Visard, P. (2015) *The Coalition's Record on Adult Social Care: Policy, spending and outcomes 2010–2015 summary.* Working paper 17, Centre for Analysis of Social Exclusion.

Burke, B. and Harrison, P. (2001) Race and racism in social work. In Davies, M. (ed.) *The Blackwell Encyclopaedia of Social Work.* Oxford: Blackwell.

Burleigh, M. (1994) *Death and Deliverance: 'Euthanasia' in Germany 1900–1945.* Cambridge: Cambridge University Press.

Burns, D., Heywood, F., Taylor, M., Wilde, P. and Wilson, M. (2004) *Making Community Participation Meaningful: A handbook for development and assessment.* Bristol: Policy Press.

Bushe, S., Kenway, P. and Aldridge, H. (2014) *How Have Low-Income Families Been Affected by Changes to Council Tax Support.* York: Joseph Rowntree Foundation.

Byrne, D. (1998) *Complexity Theory and the Social Sciences: An introduction.* London: Routledge.

Bytheway, B. (1995) *Ageism.* Buckingham: Open University Press.

Cadogan, G. and Campbell, P. (2014) *Perceptions of Crime: Findings from the 21012/13 Northern Ireland Crime Survey.* Belfast: Department of Justice Northern Ireland.

Cain, R. (2015) Work at all costs? The gendered impact of Universal Credit on lone-parent and low-paid families, http://blogs.lse.ac.uk/gender/2015/05/13/work-at-all-costs-the-gendered-impact-of-universal-credit-on-lone-parent-and-low-paid-families/ (accessed 6 June 2015).

Calder, M. and Hackett, S. (eds) (2013) *Assessment in Child Care: Using and developing frameworks for practice.* Lyme Regis: Russell House Publishing.

Cameron, C., Connelly, G. and Jackson, S. (2015) *Educating Children and Young People in Care Learning Placements and Caring Schools.* London: Jessica Kingsley Publishers.

Cameron, D. (2011) Speech on troubled families, 15 December.

Cantle, T. (2008) *Community Cohesion: A new framework for race and diversity.* Basingstoke: Palgrave Macmillan.

Carey, M. (2014) The fragmentation of social work and social care: Some ramifications and a critique. *British Journal of Social Work.* doi: 10.1093/bjsw/bcu088.

Carpenter, J. (2011) Evaluating social work education: A review of outcomes, measure, research designs and practicalities. *Social Work Education* 30, 2, 122–140.

Carrier, J. (2005) Older people, the new agenda. London: Presentation to Better Government for Older People Network.

CCETSW (1991) *Rules and Requirements for the Diploma in Social Work* (Paper 30). London: Central Council for Education and Training in Social Work.

Cemlyn, S., Greenfields, M., Burnett, S., Matthews, Z. and Whitwell, C. (2009) *Inequalities Experienced by Gypsy and Traveller Communities: A review.* London: Equality and Human Rights Commission.

Centre for Social Justice (2014) *Survival of the Fittest: Improving life chances for care leavers.* London: Centre for Social Justice.

Chalabi, M. (2014) Rising unemployment for UK's ethnic minorities: Who's affected? *Guardian,* 8 January.

Chambers, E. (2004) *Roots for Radicals: Organizing for power, action and justice.* New York and London: Continuum International Publishing.

Chaskin, R., Brown, P., Venkatesh, S. and Vidal, A. (2001) *Building Community Capacity.* New York: Aldine de Gruyter.

Chate, D. and Hazel, N. (2002) *Parenting in Poor Environments: Stress, support and coping.* London: Jessica Kingsley Publishers.

Chen, H.T. (2005) *Practical Program Evaluation: Assessing and improving program planning, implementation, and effectiveness.* London: Sage.

Chen, H. (n.d.) Theory-driven evaluation: Conceptual framework, methodology and application. Presentation, www.provalservices.net/download/Chen_presentation.pdf.

Children Society (2013) *A Good Childhood for Every Child? Child poverty in the UK.*

Citizens UK (2015) Six day training, www.citizensuk.org/six_day_training (accessed 5 January 2015).

Ciulla, J. (2004) *The Ethics of Leadership.* New York: Praeger.

Clark, C. (2000) *Social Work Ethics: Politics, principles and practice.* Basingstoke: Macmillan.

Clark, K. and Drinkwater, S. (2002) Enclaves, neighbourhood effects and employment outcomes: Ethnic minorities in England and Wales. *Journal of Population Economics* 15, 5–29.

Cohen, S. (2001) *Immigration Controls, the Family and the Welfare State.* London: Jessica Kingsley Publishers.

Coleman, J. and Hendry, L. (1999) *The Nature of Adolescence* (3rd edn). London: Routledge.

Collier, K. (2006) *Social Work with Rural Peoples* (3rd edn). Vancouver: New Star Books.

Commission for Rural Communities (2008) *Rural Financial Poverty: Good practice.* Cheltenham: Commission for Rural Communities.

Coote, A., Allen, J. and Woodhead, D. (2004) *Finding Out What Works: Building knowledge about complex, community-based initiatives.* London: King's Fund.

Coryn, C., Noakes, L., Westine, C. and Schroter, D. (2011) A systematic review of theory-driven evaluation practice from 1990 to 2009. *American Journal of Evaluation* 32, 2, 199–226.

Countryside Agency (2003) *Pockets of Deprivation: Rural initiative.* Worcester: Countryside Agency Publications.

Countryside Agency (2003) *The State of the Countryside 2003.* Worcester: Countryside Agency Publications.

Craig, G. (2001) Poverty, social work and social justice. *British Journal of Social Work* 32, 669–682.

Croucher, K. and Bevan, M. (2012) *Promoting Supportive Relationships in Housing with Care.* York: Joseph Rowntree Foundation.

Dalrymple, J. and Boylan, J. (2013) *Effective Advocacy in Social Work.* London: Sage.

Daniel, B. and Baldwin, N. (2005) The outline format for comprehensive assessment. In Taylor, J. and Daniel B. (eds) *Child Neglect.* London: Jessica Kingsley Publishers.

Das, C., O'Neill, M. and Pinkerton, J. (2015) Re-engaging with community work as a method of practice in social work: A view from Northern Ireland. *Journal of Social Work.* doi: 10.1177/1468017315569644.

Davis, A. and Wainwright, S. (2005) Combating poverty and social exclusion: Implications for social work education. *Social Work Education* 24, 3, 259–273.

Davis, F., McDonald, L. and Axford, N. (2012) Technique is not enough: A framework for ensuring that evidence-based parenting programmes are socially inclusive. British Psychological Society discussion paper.

Delbosc, A. and Currie, G. (2011) Exploring the relative influences of transport disadvantage and social exclusion on well-being. *The Journal of Transport Geography* 18, 555–562.

Dennett, A. and Stillwell, J. (2008) Population turnover and churn: Enhancing understanding of internal migration in Britain through measures of stability. *Population Trends* 134, 24–41.

Department for Children, Schools and Families (2009) *Statutory Guidance: Safeguarding children and young people from sexual exploitation.* London: Department for Children, Schools and Families.

Department for Communities and Local Government (2015) 2010 to 2015 government policy: support for families, www.gov.uk/government/publications/2010-to-2015-government-policy-support-for-families/2010-to-2015-government-policy-support-for-families (accessed 10 May 2015).

Department for Education (2012a) What to do if you suspect a child is being sexually exploited: A step-by-step guide for frontline practitioners, www.gov.uk/government/uploads/system/uploads/attachment_data/file/279511/step_by_step_guide.pdf (accessed 18 November 2014).

—— (2012b) *Looked after Children: Statistical First Release.* London: HM Government.

—— (2013) *Careers: Inspiration vision statement.* London: HM Government.

—— (2014a) Statistical Permanent and Fixed Period Exclusion in England 2012–13. London: HM Government.

—— (2014b) *Looked after Children: Statistical First Release.* London: HM Government.

—— (2014c) *Planning Transition to Adulthood for Care Leavers: Guidance to the Children Act.* London: HM Government.

—— (2015) *Exclusion from Maintained Schools, Academies and Pupil Referral Units in England and Wales: Statutory guidance for those with legal responsibilities in relation to exclusion.* London: HM Government.

Department of Environment, Farming and Rural Affairs (DEFRA) (2003) *Rural Services Standard.* London: DEFRA.

—— (2012) *Statistical Digest of Rural England 2012.* London: DEFRA.

—— (2014) *Transport and Accessibility to Services.* London: DEFRA.

Department of Health (2000a) *Framework for the Assessment of Children in Need and Their Families.* London: The Stationery Office.

—— (2003) *The Victoria Climbié Inquiry: Report of an Inquiry by Lord Laming.* London: The Stationery Office.

—— (2010) *Vision for Social Care.* London: The Stationery Office.

—— (2013) *The Adult Social Care Outcomes Framework 2014/15.* London: HM Government.

—— (2014a) *Closing the Gap: Priorities for essential change in mental health.* London: HM Government.

—— (2014b) *Care and Support Statutory Guidance under the Care Act 2014.* London: HM Government.

—— (n.d.) Capability for Work Questionnaire. London: Department for Work and Pensions.

Department for Work and Pensions (2005) *Improving Opportunity, Strengthening Society.* London: Department for Work and Pensions.

—— (2011) *Fulfilling Potential: Building a deeper understanding of disability in the UK today.* London: DWP.

—— (2014a) Disability facts and figures, www.gov.uk/government/publications/disability-facts-and-figures/disability-facts-and-figures (accessed 2 February 2015).

—— (2014b) *Jobseeker's Allowance Sanction Decisions by Jobcentre Plus Office, District and Group, 22 October 2012 to 30 June 2014.* London: Department for Work and Pensions.

—— (2015) Government to strengthen child poverty measure. Press release, Department for Work and Pensions, 1 July.

Desforges, C. and Abouchaar, A. (2003) *The Impact of Parental Involvement, Parental Support and Family Education on Pupil Achievement and Adjustment: A literature review.* Nottingham: Department for Education and Skills.

Diez Roux, A. (2001) Investigating neighborhood and area effects on health. *American Journal of Public Health* 91, 1783–1789.

Diez Roux, A. and Mair, C. (2010) Neighbourhoods and health. *Annals of the New York Academy of Sciences* 1186, 1, 125–145.

DiPrete, T. and Buchmann, C. (2013) *The Rise of Women: The growing gender gap in education and what it means for American schools.* New York: Russell Sage Foundation.

Dixon, J. and Hoatson, L. (1999) Retreat from within: Social work education's faltering commitment to community work. *Australian Social Work* 52, 2, 3–9.

Dobson, B., Middleton, S. and Beardsworth, A. (2001) *The Impact of Childhood Disability on Family Life.* York: Joseph Rowntree Foundation.

Dorling, D. (2013) Think piece in place of fear: Narrowing health inequalities, http://classonline.org.uk/docs/2013_05_Think_piece_-_In_Place_of_Fear_(Danny_Dorling).pdf.

Dorling, K., Girma, M. and Walter, N. (2012) *Refused: The experiences of women denied asylum in the UK.* London: Women for Refugee Women.

Dowling, M. (1999) *Social Workers and Poverty.* Aldershot: Ashgate.

Doyle, L. (2014) *28 Days Later: Experiences of new refugees in the UK.* London: Refugee Council.

Drew, J. (2014) Conference presentation, Coin Street Neighborhood Centre 4 Children, 26 March.

Duell, M. (2014) Revealed, the staggering scale of Britain's underclass: Half a million problem families cost the taxpayer £30 billion every year. *MailOnline*, 17 August.

Dwyer, P. and Wright, S. (2014) Universal Credit, ubiquitous conditionality and its implications for social citizenship. *Journal of Poverty and Social Justice* 22, 1, 27–35.

Ellis, A. (2002) Power and exclusion in rural community development: The case of LEADER 2 in Wales. Ph.D. thesis, University of Swansea.

Ellis, K. (2011) Street-level bureaucracy revisited: The changing face of frontline discretion in adult social care in England. *Social Policy and Administration* 45, 3, 221–244.

Emerson, E., Graham, H., McCulloch, A., Blacher, J. and Llewellyn, G. (2009) The social context of parenting 3-year-old children with developmental delay in the UK. *Child Care Health and Development* 35, 1, 63–70.

Erikson, E. (1965) *Childhood and Society*. London: Penguin.

Evans, R. and Holland, S. (2012) Community parenting. *Families, Relationships and Societies* 1, 2, 173–190.

Evans, T. (2013) Organisational rules and discretion in adult social work. *British Journal of Social Work* 43, 739–758.

Ewing, R., Govekar, M., Govekar, P. and Rishi, M. (2002) Economics, market segmentation and recruiting: Targeting your promotion to volunteers' needs. *Journal of Nonprofit and Public Sector Marketing* 10, 63–96.

Falkingham, J., Evandrou, M., McGowan, T., Bell, D. and Bowes, A. (2010) *Demographic Issues, Projections and Trends: Older people with high support needs in the UK*. Southampton: Centre for Population Change, University of Southampton.

Farver, J. and Natera, L. (2000) Effects of neighborhood violence on preschoolers' social function with peers. *International Perspectives on Child and Adolescent Mental Health*, Volume 1: Proceedings of the First International Conference, 41–57.

Featherstone, B., Morris, K. and White, S. (2014) A marriage made in Hell: Early intervention meets child protection. *British Journal of Social Work* 44, 1735–1749.

Feinstein, L., Duckworth, K. and Sabates, R. (2008) *Education and the Family: Passing success across the generations*. Abingdon: Routledge.

Ferguson, R. and Stoutland, S. (1999) Reconceiving the community development field. In Ferguson, R. and Dickens, W. (eds) *Urban Problems and Community Development*, Washington, DC: The Brookings Institution.

Field, F. (2010) *The Foundation Years: Preventing poor children becoming poor adults: Report of the independent review on poverty and life chances*. London: HM Government.

Fine, C. (2010) *Delusions of Gender: The real science behind sex differences*. London: Icon.

Finn, D. and Goodship, J. (2014) *Take-Up of Benefits and Poverty: An evidence and policy review*. London: Centre for Economic and Social Inclusion.

Fish, J. (2010) Conceptualising social exclusion and LGBT people: The implication for promoting equity in nursing policy and practice. *Journal of Nursing Research* 15, 4, 303–312.

Folbre, N. (2001) *The Invisible Heart: Economics and family values*. New York: The New Press.

Frechtling, J. (2007) *Logic Modeling Methods in Program Evaluation*. San Francisco: John Wiley & Sons.

Freud, E. (2012) Ella's story. In Dorling, K., Girma, M. and Walter, N., *Refused: The experiences of women denied asylum in the UK*. London: Women for Refugee Women.

Friedman, M. (1962) *Capitalism and Freedom*. Chicago: Chicago University Press.

Furlong, A. and Cartmel, F. (2004) *Vulnerable Young Men in Fragile Labour Markets: Employment, unemployment and the search for long-term security*. York: Joseph Rowntree Foundation.

—— (2007) *Young People and Social Change: New perspectives*. Buckingham: Open University Press.

Gadd, D. and Dixon, B. (2011) *Losing the Race: Thinking psychosocially about racially motivated crime* (Exploring Psycho-Social Studies). London: Karnac Books.

Garrett, P. (2002) Social work and the just society: Diversity, difference and the sequestration of poverty. *Journal of Social Work* 2, 2, 187–210.

Gilbert, R., Widom, C.S., Brown, K., Fergusson, D., Webb, E. and Janson, S. (2009) Burden and consequences of child maltreatment in high-income countries. *The Lancet* 373, 68–81.

Gill, O. and Jack, J. (2012) *The Child and Family in Context: Developing ecological practice in disadvantaged communities*. Lyme Regis: Russell House Publishing.

Gilligan, P. (2007) Well motivated reformists or nascent radicals: How do applicants to the degree in social work see social problems, their origins and solutions? *British Journal of Social Work* 37, 735–760.

Gilligan, R. (2008) Resilience and young people leaving care. *Child Care in Practice* 14, 1.

Girl Guiding (2012) *Girls' Attitudes Survey 2012*. London: The Guide Association.

Glendinning, C., Powell, M. and Rummery K. (2002) *Partnerships, New Labour and the Governance of Welfare*. Bristol: Policy Press.

Glendinning, C., Challis, D., Fernández, J.-L., Jacobs, S., Jones, K., Knapp, M., Manthorpe, J., Moran, N., Netten, A., Steven, M. and Wilberforce, M. (2008) *Evaluation of the Individual Budgets Pilot Programme: Final report*. York: Social Policy Research Unit, University of York.

Golden, M., Samuels, M. and Southall, D. (2003) How to distinguish between neglect and deprivational abuse. *Archives of Disease in Childhood* 88, 2, 105–107.

Goodley, D. (2005) Empowerment, self-advocacy and resilience. *Journal of Intellectual Disabilities* 9, 4, 333–343.

Gove, M. (2013) Getting it right for children in need. Speech to the NSPCC, 12 November.

Graham, H. (2013) Lone parents, employment and well-being: What does the evidence tell us? Presentation, Employment Research Institute, Edinburgh Napier University.

Granovetter, M. (1973) The strength of weak ties hypothesis. *American Journal of Sociology* 78, 8, 1360–1380.

Gridley, N., Hutchings, J. and Baker-Henningham, H. (2013) Associations between socio-economic disadvantage and parenting behaviours. *Journal of Children's Services* 8, 4, 254–263.

Griffiths, C. (2014) Civilised communities. *British Journal of Criminology* 54, 1109–1128.

Hacker, J. (2009) *The Great Risk Shift: The new economic insecurity and decline of the American dream?* Oxford: Oxford University Press.

Hamer, C. (2006) Parents in partnership with practitioners creating a reality. University of East London.

Harris, I. (1995) *Messages Men Hear: Constructing masculinities*. London: Taylor & Francis.

Hatton, C., Collins, M., Welch, V., Robertson, J., Emerson, E., Langer, S. and Wells, E. (2011) *The Impact of Short Breaks on Families with a Disabled Child over Time* (Department for Education Research Report). London: Department for Education.

Hayes, D. and Humphries, B. (2004) *Social Work, Immigration and Asylum: Debates, Dilemmas and Ethical Issues for Social Work and Social Care Practice*. London: Jessica Kingsley Publishers.

Heenan, D. (2006) The factors influencing access to health and social care in the farming communities of County Down, Northern Ireland. *Ageing and Society* 26, 373–391.

Hemingway, A. and Jack, E. (2013) Reducing social isolation and promoting well-being in older people. *Quality in Ageing and Older Adults* 14, 1, 25–35.

Hemmings, C. and Kabesh, A. (2013) The feminist subject of agency: Recognition and affect in encounters with 'the Other'. In Madhok, S., Phillips, A. and Wilson, K. (eds) *Gender, Agency, and Coercion*. Basingstoke: Palgrave Macmillan.

Hetherington, P. (2009) Uphill strugglers. *Guardian*, 11 February.

Hillman, J. and Williams, T. (2015) *Early Years Education and Childcare: Lessons from evidence and future priorities*. London: Nuffield Foundation.

Hills, J. (2015) *Falling Behind, Getting Ahead: The changing structure of inequality in the UK, 2007–2013* (Research Report 5). London: Centre for Analysis of Social Exclusion.

Hirsch, D. (2008) *Estimating the Costs of Child Poverty*. York: Joseph Rowntree Foundation.

HM Government (2012) *Social Justice: Transforming lives* (Cmnd 8314). London: The Stationery Office.

—— (2013) *Universal Credit Regulations 2013*. London: The Stationery Office.

HM Inspectorate of Prisons (2011) *The Care of Looked After Children in Custody: A short thematic review*. London: HMIP.

HMRC (2013) *Child Benefit, Child Tax Credit and Working Tax Credit: Take-up rates: 2011–12*. London: Her Majesty's Revenue and Customs.

Holland, S., Burgess, S., Grogan-Kaylor, A. and Delva, J. (2011) Understanding neighbourhoods, communities and environments: New approaches for social work research. *British Journal of Social Work* 41, 689–707.

Hollister, R. (2007) Measuring the impact of community development financial institutions' activities. In Rubin, J. (ed.) *Financing Low Income Communities*. New York: Russell Sage Foundation.

Hollywood, E., Egdell, V. and McQuaid, R. (2012) Addressing the issue of disadvantaged youth seeking work. *Social Work and Society* 10, 1.

Home Office (2012) *Putting Victims First: More effective responses to anti-social behaviour*. London: The Stationery Office.

House of Commons (2014) Benefits sanctions policy beyond the Oakley Review. Work and Pensions Select Committee, 24 March.

Howarth, J. (2007) The missing assessment domain: Personal, professional and organizational factors influencing professional judgements when identifying and referring child neglect. *British Journal of Social Work* 37, 1285–1303.

Huari, H. and Cameron, C. (2014) England: A targeted approach. In Jackson, S. and Cameron, C. (eds) *Improving Access to Further and Higher Education for Young People in Public Care*. London: Jessica Kingsley Publishers.

Hughes, A. (n.d.) Lone parents and paid work: Case studies from rural England (End of award report). Swindon: ESRC.

—— (2004) Geographies of invisibility: The 'hidden' lives of rural lone parents. In Holloway, L. and Kneafsey, M. (eds) *Geographies of Rural Cultures and Societies*. Farnham: Ashgate.

Hughes, M. and Traynor, T. (2000) Reconciling process and outcome in evaluating community initiatives. *Evaluation* 6, 1, 37–49.

Institute of Fiscal Studies (2014) *Welfare Reform and Work Incentives in the UK*. London: IFS.

Jack, G. (2000) Ecological perspectives in assessing children and families. In Howarth, J. (ed.) *The Child's World: Assessing children in need*. London: Jessica Kingsley Publishers.

Jack, G. and Gill, O. (2010) The role of communities in safeguarding children and young people. *Child Abuse Review* 19, 82–96.

Jackson, C. (2003). Motives for 'laddishness' at school: Fear of failure and fear of the 'feminine'. *British Educational Research Journal* 29, 4, 583–598.

Jackson, S. and Cameron, C. (2014) *Improving Access to Further and Higher Education for Young People in Public Care*. London: Jessica Kingsley Publishers.

Jacobs, S., Abell, J., Steven, M., Wilberforce, M., Challis, D., Manthorpe, J., Fernandez, J.-L., Glendinning, C., Jones, K., Knapp, M., Moran, N. and Netten, A. (2013) The personalization of care services and the early impact on staff activity patterns. *Journal of Social Work* 13, 2, 141–163.

Jamieson, L. and Groves, L. (2008) *Drivers of Youth Out-Migration from Rural Scotland*. Edinburgh: Scottish Government Social Research.

Jay, A. (2014). *Independent Inquiry into Sexual Exploitation in Rotherham 1997–2013*. Rotherham Borough Council.

Jivraj, S. and Khan, O. (2013) Ethnicity and deprivation in England: How likely are ethnic minorities to live in deprived neighbourhoods? (briefing paper). Manchester: Centre on Dynamics of Ethnicity.

Joint Committee on Human Rights (2013) *Human Rights of Unaccompanied Migrant Children and Young People in the UK*. London: House of Commons and House of Lords.

Jones, C. (2005) The neo-liberal assault: Voices from the front line of British state social work. In Ferguson, I., Lavalette, M. and Whitmore, E. (eds) *Globalisation, Global Justice and Social Work*. London: Routledge.

Jones, K., Daley, D., Hutchings, J., Bywater, T. and Eames, C. (2008) Efficacy of the Incredible Years Programme as an early intervention for children with conduct problems and ADHD: Long-term follow-up. *Child Care Health Development* 34, 3, 380–390.

Julkunen, I. (2011) Critical elements in evaluating and developing practice in social work: An exploratory overview. *Social Work and Social Science Review* 15, 1, 74–91.

Kaner, S., Lind, L., Toldi, C., Fisk, S. and Berger, D. (1996) *Facilitators Guide to Participatory Decision-Making*. Gabriola Island, British Columbia: New Society Publishers.

Keating, N., Orfinowski, P., Wenger, C., Fast, J. and Derksen, L. (2003) Understanding the caring capacity of informal networks of frail seniors: A case for care networks. *Ageing and Society* 23, 115–127.

Kelly, R. and Philpott, S. (2003) *Community Cohesion Moving Bradford Forward: Lessons from Northern Ireland*. Bradford: University of Bradford.

Kenyon, S. (2011) Transport and social exclusion: Access to higher education in the UK policy context. *Journal of Transport Geography* 19, 763–771.

Kohli, R. (2007) *Social Work with Unaccompanied Asylum-Seeking Children*. Basingstoke: Palgrave Macmillan.

Kotecha, K., Arthur, S. and Coutinho, S. (n.d.) *Understanding the Relationship between Pensioner Poverty and Material Deprivation* (Research report 827). London: Department for Work and Pensions.

Krugman, P. (2013) How the case for austerity has crumbled. *New York Review of Books*, 6 June.

—— (2015) This snookered isle: Britain's terrible, no-good economic discourse. *New York Times*, 23 March.

Krumer-Nevo, M., Weiss-Gal, I. and Levin, L. (2011) Searching for poverty-aware social work: Discourse analysis of job descriptions. *Journal of Social Policy* 40, 2, 313–332.

Kubisch, A. and Stone, R. (2001) Comprehensive community initiatives: The American experience. In Pierson, J. and Smith, J. (eds) *Rebuilding Community: The policy and practice of urban regeneration*. Basingstoke: Palgrave Macmillan.

Lalani, M., Metcalf, H., Tufekci, L., Corley, A., Rolfe, H. and George, A. (2014) *How Place Influences Employment Outcomes for Ethnic Minorities*. York: Joseph Rowntree Foundation.

Lambie-Mumford, H. (2014) *Food Bank Provision and Welfare Reform in the UK*. Sheffield: University of Sheffield.

Larner, W. (2006) Global governance and local policy partnerships. In Marston, G. and McDonald, C. (eds) *Analysing Social Policy: A governmental approach*. Cheltenham: Edward Elgar.

Lawrence, K. (2001) Structural racism and comprehensive community initiatives. In Pierson, J. and Smith, J. (eds) *Rebuilding Community: Policy and practice of urban regeneration*. Basingstoke: Palgrave Macmillan.

Lea, J. (2000) The Macpherson Report and the question of institutional racism. *The Howard Journal* 39, 3, 219–233.

Levitas, R. (2005) *The Inclusive Society? Social exclusion and New Labour*. Basingstoke: Macmillan.

—— (2012) There may be 'trouble' ahead: What we know about those 120,000 'troubled' families. PSE UK.

Leyshon, M. (2003) Youth identity, culture and marginalisation in the countryside. Ph.D. thesis, University of Exeter, Department of Geography.

Lipset, S. (1996) *American Exceptionalism*. New York: Norton.

Litchfield, P. (2014) An independent review of the Work Capability Assessment, www.gov.uk/government/uploads/system/uploads/attachment_data/file/380027/wca-fifth-independent-review.pdf.

Livingston, M., Bailey, N. and Kearns, A. (2008) *People's Attachment to Place: The influence of neighbourhood deprivation*. Coventry: Chartered Institute of Housing.

Lloyd, E. and Penn, H. (2013) *Childcare Markets: Can they deliver an equitable service?* Bristol: Policy Press.

London Councils (2014) *Anti-Social Behaviour and Mental Health*. London: London Councils.

Loopstra, R., Reeves, A., McKee, D. and Stuckler, D. (2015) Do punitive approaches to unemployment benefit recipients increase welfare exits and employment? A cross-area analysis of UK sanctioning reforms. Oxford: University of Oxford, Department of Sociology.

Luxmoore, N. (2000) *Listening to Young People in School, Youth Work and Counselling*. London: Jessica Kingsley Publishers.

—— (2008) *Feeling Like Crap: Young people and the meaning of self-esteem*. London: Jessica Kingsley Publishers.

Lymbery, M. (2014) Understanding personalisation: Implications for social work. *Journal of Social Work* 14, 3, 295–312.

MacDonald, H. and Callery, P. (2008) Parenting children requiring complex care: A journey through time. *Child Care, Health and Development* 34, 2, 207–213.

MacInnes, T., Aldridge, H., Bushe, S., Tinson, A. and Born, T. (2014) *Monitoring Poverty and Social Exclusion*. York: Joseph Rowntree Foundation and New Policy Institute.

Mack, J., Lansley, S., Nandy, S. and Pantazis, C. (2013) Attitudes to necessities in the PSE 2012 survey: Are minimum standards becoming less generous? PSE UK.

Macpherson, Sir William (1999) *The Stephen Lawrence Inquiry* (Cm 4262-I). London: The Stationery Office.

Madge, N., Burton, S., Howell, S. and Hearn, B. (2000) *9–13: The forgotten years?* London: National Children's Bureau.

Manthorpe, J. and Samsi, K. (2013) 'Inherently risky?' Personal budgets for people with dementia and the risks of financial abuse: Findings from an interview-based study with adult safeguarding coordinators. *British Journal of Social Work* 43, 889–903.

Manthorpe, J., Harris, J., Hussein, S., Cornes, M. and Moriarty, J. (2014) *Evaluation of the Social Work Practices with Adults Pilots* (Final Report). London: King's College, Social Care Workforce Research Unit.

Mantle, G. and Backwith, D. (2010) Poverty and social work. *British Journal of Social Work* 40, 2380–2397.

Marshall, T.H. (1950) *Citizenship and Social Class and Other Essays*. Cambridge: Cambridge University Press.

McConkey, R. (2011) *Working Outside the Box: An evaluation of short breaks and intensive support services to families and disabled young people whose behavior is severely challenging*. Watford: Action for Children.

McDowell, K. (2015) Personal communication with the author.

McGhee, D. (2003) Moving to 'our' common ground – a critical examination of community cohesion discourse in twenty-first century Britain. *Sociological Review* 51, 3, 376–404.

McLeod, E. and Bywaters, P. (2000) *Social Work, Health and Equality*. London: Routledge.

McLeod, E., Bywaters, P., Tanner, D. and Hirsch, M. (2008) For the sake of their health: Older service users' requirements for social care to facilitate access to social networks following hospital discharge. *British Journal of Social Work* 38, 1, 73–90.

Melrose, M. (2013) Young people and sexual exploitation: A critical discourse analysis. In Melrose, M. and Pearce, J. (eds) *Critical Perspectives on Child Sexual Exploitation and Related Trafficking*. Basingstoke: Palgrave Macmillan.

Mendes, P. (2009) Teaching community development to social work students: A critical reflection. *Community Development Journal* 44, 2, 248–262.

Mental Health Foundation (2013) *The Lonely Society?* www.mentalhealth.org.uk/content/assets/pdf/publications/the_lonely_society_report.pdf (accessed 9 September 2014).

Milbourne, P. and Doheny, S. (2012) Older people and poverty in rural Britain: Material hardships, cultural denials and social inclusions. *Journal of Rural Studies* 28, 389–397.

Millie, A., Jacobson, J., McDonald, E. and Hough, M. (2005) *Anti-Social Behaviour Strategies: Finding a balance.* Bristol: Policy Press.

Mitchell, G. and Campbell, L. (2011) The social economy of excluded families. *Child and Family Social Work* 16, 422–433.

Modood, T. (2007) *Multiculturalism.* Cambridge: Polity Press.

Mohan, J. and Bulloch, S. (2012) The idea of a 'civic core': What are the overlaps between charitable giving, volunteering, and civic participation in England and Wales? (TSRC Briefing Paper 73). Birmingham: Third Sector Research Centre.

Monnickendam, M., Katz, C. and Monnickendam, M.S. (2010) Social workers serving poor clients: Perception of poverty and service policy. *British Journal of Social Work* 40, 911–927.

Morris, K. (2006) Camden Family Group Conference Service: An evaluation of service outcomes. London Borough of Camden.

——— Thinking family? The complexities for family engagement in care and protection. *British Journal of Social Work* 42, 906–920.

Morris, K. and Barnes, M. (2008) Prevention and social exclusion: New understanding for policy and practice. *British Journal of Social Work* 38, 6, 1194–1211.

Muir, K. and Strnadova, I. (2014) Whose responsibility? Resilience in families of children with development disabilities. *Disability and Society* 29, 6, 922–937.

Mullainathan, S. and Shafir, E. (2014) *Scarcity: The new science of having less and how it defines our lives.* New York: Picador.

Murray, C. (1996) Underclass: The crisis deepens. In Lister, R. (ed.) *Charles Murray and the Underclass: The developing debate.* London: Institute of Economic Affairs.

NAO COMPASS (2014) *Contracts for the Provision of Accommodation for Asylum Seekers.* London: National Audit Office.

National Association of Welfare Rights Advisers (2014) Response to the call for information: Independent review of Job Seeker's Allowance sanctions, www.nawra.org.uk/wordpress/wordpress/wp-content/uploads/2012/03/Independent-review-of-sanctions-January-20141.pdf.

National Audit Office (2015) *Care Leavers' Transition to Adulthood.* London: Department for Education.

National Council for Voluntary Organisations (2011) *Participation: Trends, facts and figures.* London: NCVO.

NESS (2012) *The Impact of Sure Start Local Programmes on Seven Year Olds and Their Families.* London: Department for Education.

Netten, A., Forder, J. and Shapiro, J. (2006) *Measuring Personal Social Service Outputs for National Accounts: Services for older people.* Manchester: Personal Social Services Research Unit.

Netten, A., Jones, K., Knapp, M., Fernandez, J.-L., Challis, D., Glendinning, C., Jacobs, S., Manthorpe, J., Moran, N., Stevens, M. and Wilberforce, M. (2012) Personalisation through Individual Budgets: Does it work and for whom? *British Journal of Social Work* 42, 1556–1573.

Nixon, J. (2007) Deconstructing 'problem' researchers and 'problem' families: A rejoinder to Garrett. *Critical Social Policy* 27, 4, 546–564.

Nozick, R. (1974) *Anarchy, State and Utopia.* London: Wiley-Blackwell.

O'Connor, A. (2001) *Poverty Knowledge: Social science, social policy, and the poor in twentieth-century U.S. history.* Princeton, NJ: Princeton University Press.

Oliver, M. (1990). *The Politics of Disablement.* Basingstoke: Macmillan.

Oliver, M. and Sapey, B. (2006) *Social Work with Disabled People* (3rd revised edn). Basingstoke: Palgrave Macmillan.

Orenstein, P. (2012) *Cinderella Ate My Daughter: Dispatches from the front lines of the new girlie-girl culture.* London: Harper Paperbacks.

O'Rourke, D. (2015) A new way of working is transforming mental health services in Lambeth. *Guardian*, 15 April.

Ousley, H. (2001) *Community Pride, Not Prejudice*. Bradford: Bradford City Council.

Palmer, G., MacInnes, T. and Kenway, P. (2006) *Monitoring Poverty and Social Exclusion 2006*. London: New Policy Institute.

—— (2008) *Monitoring Poverty and Social Exclusion 2008*. York: Joseph Rowntree Foundation and New Policy Institute.

Parekh, B. (2000) *The Future of Multi-Ethnic Britain: The Parekh Report*. London: Profile Books.

Parkinson, G. (1970) I give them money. In Fitzgerald *et al.* (eds) (1977) *Welfare in Action*. London: Routledge & Kegan Paul.

Patterson, G. (1985) *Anti-Social Boys*. Eugene, OR: Castalia Publishing.

Paugam, S. (1993) *L'exclusion: L'état des savoirs*. Paris: La Découverte.

Pawson, R. and Tilley, N. (1997) *Realistic Evaluation*. London: Sage.

Pearson, G. (1989) Social work and unemployment. In Langan, M. and Lee, P. (eds) *Radical Social Work Today*. London: Unwin Hyman.

Penketh, L. (2001) *Tackling Institutional Racism: Anti-racist policies and social work education and training*. Bristol: Policy Press.

Phillips, M. (2011) Material, cultural, moral and emotional inscriptions of class and gender: Impressions from gentrified rural England. In Pini, B. and Leach, B. (eds) *Reshaping Gender and Class in Rural Spaces*. Aldershot: Ashgate.

Pierson, J. (2011) *Understanding Social Work: History and context*. Maidenhead: Open University Press.

Pilling, S., Gould, N., Whittington, C., Taylor, C. and Scott, S. (2013) Recognition, intervention and management of antisocial behavior and conduct disorders in children and young people: Summary of NICE-SCIE guidance. *British Medical Journal* 346, 1298.

Pitts, J. (2014) If only someone had listened. Conference presentation, Coin Street Neighborhood Centre 4 Children, 26 March.

Poppendieck, J. (1999) *Sweet Charity? Emergency food and the end of entitlement*. London: Penguin.

Power, A. (1997) *Estates on the Edge*. Basingstoke: Palgrave Macmillan.

Power, A. and Mumford, K. (1999) *The Slow Death of Great Cities? Urban abandonment or urban renaissance*. York: Joseph Rowntree Foundation.

Power, A. and Tunstall, R. (1997) *Dangerous Disorder: Riots and violent disturbances in thirteen areas of Britain, 1991–92*. York: Joseph Rowntree Foundation.

Preston, J. and Rajé, F. (2007) Accessibility, mobility and transport-related social exclusion. *Journal of Transport Geography* 15, 151–160.

Pugh, R. (2003) Considering the countryside: Is there a case for rural social work? *British Journal of Social Work* 33, 67–85.

—— (2007) Dual relationships: Personal and professional boundaries in rural social work. *British Journal of Social Work* 37, 8, 1405–1423.

Putnam, R. (2001) *Bowling Alone: The collapse and revival of American community*. London: Simon & Shuster.

—— (2007) *E pluribus unum*: Diversity and community in the twenty-first century (The 2006 Johan Skytte Prize lecture). *Scandinavian Political Studies* 30, 137–174.

Rabiee, P. (2013) Exploring the relationships between choice and independence: Experiences of disabled and older people. *British Journal of Social Work* 43, 872–888.

Rabiee, P. and Glendinning, C. (2014) Choice and control for older people using home care services: How far have council-managed personal budgets helped? *Quality in Ageing and Older Adults* 15, 4, 210–219.

Rabin, S. and McKenzie, D. (2014) *A Better Offer: The future of volunteering in an ageing society*. London: Commission on the Voluntary Sector and Ageing.

Rawls, J. (1971) *A Theory of Justice*. Cambridge, MA: Harvard University Press.

Reimer, B. (2006) The rural context of community development in Canada. *Journal of Rural and Community Development* 1, 155–175.

Riley, K.A. and Docking, J. (2004) Voices of disaffected pupils: Implications for policy and practice. *British Journal of Educational Studies* 52, 2, 166–179.

Riots Communities and Victims Panel (2012) *After the Riots: The final report*. London: Riots Communities and Victims Panel.

Roberts, R. (1973) *The Classic Slum*. London: Penguin.

Robinson, K. (2014) Voices from the frontline: Social work with refugees and asylum seekers in Australia and the UK. *British Journal of Social Work* 44, 6, 1602–1620.

Rossi, P., Lipsey, M. and Freeman, H. (2003) *Evaluation: A systematic approach* (7th edn). London: Sage.

Rural Poverty and Inclusion Working Group (2001) *Poverty and Social Exclusion in Rural Scotland*. Edinburgh: The Scottish Executive.

Rutter, M., Giller, H. and Hagell, A. (1998) *Anti-Social Behavior by Young People*. Cambridge: Cambridge University Press.

Sabel, C. (1993) Studied trust: Building new forms of cooperation in a volatile economy. *Human Relations* 46, 1133–1170.

Sammons, P., Sylva, K., Melhuish, E., Sirag-Blatchford, I. and Taggart, B. (eds) (2010) *Early Childhood Matters: Evidence from the Effective Pre-school and Primary Education project*. Abingdon: Routledge.

Sampson, R. (1999) What 'community' supplies. In Ferguson, R. and Dickens, W. (eds) *Urban Problems and Community Development*. Washington, DC: The Brookings Institution.

—— (2013) *The Great American City: Chicago and the enduring neighborhood effect*. Chicago: University of Chicago Press.

Sampson, R., Morenoff, J. and Gannon-Rowley, T. (2002) Assessing 'neighborhood effects': Social processes and new directions in research. *Annual Review of Sociology* 28, 443–478.

Sandel, M. (2009) *Justice: What's the right thing to do?* London: Penguin.

—— (2013) *What Money Can't Buy: The moral limits of markets*. London: Penguin.

Scharf, T., Phillipson, C. and Smith, E. (2005) *Multiple Exclusion and Quality of Life amongst Excluded Older People in Disadvantaged Neighbourhoods*. London: Office of Deputy Prime Minister.

Schier, S. (2000) *By Invitation Only*. Pittsburgh: University of Pittsburgh Press.

Schildrick, T., MacDonald, R., Webster, C. and Garthwaite, K. (2012) *Poverty and Insecurity: Life in low-pay, no-pay Britain*. Bristol: Policy Press.

Schlozman, K., Verba, S. and Brady, H. (2013) *The Unheavenly Chorus: Unequal political voice and the broken promise of American democracy*. London: Princeton University Press.

Schmid, K., Al Ramiah, A. and Hewstone, M. (2014) Neighborhood ethnic diversity and trust: The role of the intergroup contact and perceived threat. *Psychological Science* 25, 3, 665–674.

Scope (2015) *Enabling Work*.

Scottish Executive (2001) *Poverty and Social Exclusion in Rural Scotland: A report by the Rural Poverty and Inclusion Working Group*. Edinburgh: The Scottish Executive.

Sellers, B. and Arrigo, B. (2009) Adolescent transfer, developmental maturity, and adjudicative competence: An ethical and justice policy inquiry. *Journal of Criminal Law and Criminology* 99, 3, 435–488.

Sen, A. (1983) *Poverty and Famines: An essay on entitlement and deprivation*. Oxford: Oxford University Press.

Sennett, R. (1998) *The Corrosion of Character: The personal consequences of work in the new capitalism*. London: W.W. Norton.

Shakespeare, T. and Watson, N. (2002) The social model of disability: An outdated ideology? *Research in Social Science and Disability* 2, 9–28.

Shaw, I. (2011) *Evaluating in Practice*. Farnham: Ashgate.

Sheldon, B. and Chilvers, R. (2001) *Evidence-Based Social Care: A study of prospects and problems*. Lyme Regis: Russell House.

Shiner, M., Young, T., Newburn, T. and Groben, S. (2004) Mentoring disaffected young people: An evaluation of Mentoring Plus. York: Joseph Rowntree Foundation.

Shucksmith, M. (2000) *Exclusive Countryside? Social inclusion and regeneration in rural Britain*. York: Joseph Rowntree Foundation.

—— (2002) *Social Exclusion in Rural Areas: A review of recent research*. Aberdeen: Arkleton Centre for Rural Development Research, University of Aberdeen.

—— (2004) *Social Exclusion in Rural Areas: A review of recent research*. Aberdeen: University of Aberdeen.

—— (2012) Class, power and inequality in rural areas: Beyond social exclusion? *Sociologia Ruralis* 52, 4, 377–397.

Siddique, H. (2014) Work capability assessment system at 'virtual collapse' says judge. *Guardian*, 11 June.

Silver, H. and Miller, S. (2003). Social exclusion: The European approach to social disadvantage. *Indicators* 2, 2, 5–21.

Sinclair, D. and Watson, J. (2014) *Making Our Communities Ready for Ageing: A call to action*. London: Age UK.

Sipal, R., Schuengel, C., Voorman, J., Van Eck, M. and Becher, J. (2009) Course of behaviour problems of children with cerebral palsy: The role of parental stress and support. *Child Care, Health and Development* 36, 1, 74–84.

Sluzki, C. (2000) Social networks and the elderly: Conceptual and clinical issues, and a family consultation. *Family Process* 39, 3, 271–278.

Smale, G. (1998) *Managing Change Through Innovation*. London: The Stationery Office.

Smale, G., Tuson, G., Biehal, N. and Marsh, P. (1993) *Empowerment, Assessment, Care Management and the Skilled Worker*. London: HMSO.

Smale, G., Tuson, G. and Statham, D. (2000) *Social Work and Social Problems: Working towards social inclusion and social change*. Basingstoke: Macmillan.

Social Care Institute of Excellence (2014) *Keeping Personal Budgets Personal: Learning from the experiences of older people, people with mental health problems and their carers* (Report 40). London: Social Care Institute of Excellence.

Social Exclusion Task Force (2004) *Tackling Social Exclusion: Taking stock and looking to the future*. London: Office of the Deputy Prime Minister.

—— (2008) *Think Family: Improving the life chances of families at risk*. London: Cabinet Office.

Solnit, R. (2014) *Men Explain Things to Me and Other Essays*. London: Granta.

Spencer, N. and Baldwin, N. (2005) Economic, cultural, and social contexts of neglect. In Taylor, J. and Daniel, B. (eds) *Child Neglect: Practice issues for health and social care*. London: Jessica Kingsley Publishers.

Squires, P. (2008) *ASBO Nation: The criminalisation of nuisance*. Bristol: Policy Press.

Stalker, K. and Moscardini, L. (2012) *A Critical Review and Analysis of Current Research and Policy Relating to Disabled Children and Young People in Scotland*. A report to Scotland's Commissioner for Children and Young People. Strathclyde: University of Strathclyde.

Stein, M. (2010) *Increasing the Number of Care Leavers in 'Settled, Safe Accommodation'*. Glasgow: Centre for Excellence and Outcomes in Children and Young People's Services.

—— (2012) *Young People Leaving Care: Supporting pathways to adulthood*. London: Jessica Kingsley Publishers.

—— (2014) How does care leaver support in the UK compare with the rest of the world? *Community Care*, 23 October.

Stokes, J. and Schmidt, G. (2011) Race, poverty and child protection decision making. *British Journal of Social Work* 41, 1105–1121.

Stone, R. and Butler, B. (2000) *Core Issues in Comprehensive Community Building Initiatives: Exploring power and 'race'*. Chicago: Chapin Hall Centre for Children, University of Chicago.

Storey, D. (2013) 'New' migrants in the British countryside. *Journal of Rural and Community Development* 8, 3, 291–302.

Stout, J. (2010) *Blessed Are the Organized Grassroots Democracy in America*. London: Princeton University Press.

Sun, A. (2001) Perceptions among social work and non-social work students concerning causes of poverty. *Journal of Social Work Education* 37, 161–173.

Thomas, M. (2015) personal communication.

Thompson, E. (1977) *Whigs and Hunters: Origins of the Black Act*. London: Peregrine.

Tilley, N. (2000) Realist evaluation: An overview. Conference of the Danish Evaluation Society, http://healthimpactassessment.pbworks.com/f/Realistic+evaluation+an+overview+-+UoNT+England+-+2000.pdf.

Tilly, C. (1999) *Durable Inequality*. London: University of California Press.

Tönnies, F. (2001) *Community and Civil Society*. Cambridge: Cambridge University Press (first published 1887).

Townsend, P. (1979) *Poverty in the United Kingdom*. London: Penguin.

—— (2010) The meaning of poverty. *The British Journal of Sociology: The BJS: Shaping Sociology Over 60 Years* (pp. 85–102). (Originally published in 1962 in *British Journal of Sociology* 13, 3, 210–227.)

Trussell Trust (2014) *UK Foodbank Network*. Salisbury, UK.

Tunstall, R. (2009) *Communities in Recession: The impact on deprived neighbourhoods*. York: Joseph Rowntree Foundation.

Turbett, C. (2006) Rural social work in Scotland and Eastern Canada: A comparison between the experience of practitioners in remote communities. *International Social Work* 49, 5, 583–594.

Turney, D., Platt, D., Selwyn, J. and Farmer, E. (2011) *Social Work Assessment of Children in Need: What do we know? Messages from research*. London: Department for Education.

Turney, D., Platt, D., Selwyn, J. and Farmer, E. (2012) *Improving Child and Family Assessments: Turning research into practice*. London: Jessica Kingsley Publishers.

Varshney, A. (2002) *Ethnic Conflict and Civic Life: Hindus and Muslims in India*. London: Yale University Press.

Waldfogel, J. (2000). What we know and don't know about the state of child protective service system and the links between poverty and child maltreatment. Remarks for Joint Center for Poverty Research Congressional Research Briefing on 'Child welfare and child protection: Current research and policy implications'. Washington, DC, 14 September.

—— (2010) *Britain's War on Poverty*. New York: Russell Sage Foundation.

Walker, R. (2014) *The Shame of Poverty*. Oxford: Oxford University Press.

Ward, C. (2012) *Perspectives on Ageing with a Learning Disability*. York: Joseph Rowntree Foundation.

Wastell, D. and White, S. (2012) Blinded by neuroscience: Social policy, the family and the infant brain. *Families, Relationships and Societies* 1, 3, 397–414.

Watts, B., Fitzpatrick, S., Bramley, G. and Watkins, D. (2014) *Welfare Sanctions and Conditionality in the UK*. York: Joseph Rowntree Foundation.

Weatherburn, D. and Lind, B. (2001) *Delinquent-Prone Communities*. Cambridge: Cambridge University Press.

Webster, D. (2015) Benefit sanctions: Britain's secret penal system. London: Centre for Crime and Justice Studies, www.crimeandjustice.org.uk/resources/benefit-sanctions-britains-secret-penal-systemacc (accessed 30 March 2015).

Welsh Assembly (2004) *Settlements, Services and Access: The development of policies to promote accessibility in rural areas in Great Britain*. Cardiff: Welsh Assembly.

Wenger, C. (1997) Social networks and the prediction of elderly people at risk. *Ageing and Mental Health* 1, 311–320.

Wilkinson, D. and Applebee, E. (1999) *Implementing Holistic Government: Joined-up action on the ground*. London: Demos.

Wilkinson, R. and Pickett, K. (2010) *The Spirit Level: Why equality is better for everyone.* London: Penguin.

Wilson, W. (1996) *When Work Disappears: The world of the new urban poor.* New York: Alfred Knopf.

Wilson, C., Philpot, T. and Hanvey, S. (2011) *A Community-Based Approach to the Reduction of Sexual Reoffending: Circles of support and accountability.* London: Jessica Kingsley Publishers.

Winterbotham, M., Vivian, D., Shury, J. and Davies, B. (2014) *UK Commission's Employer Skills Survey 2013: UK results.* London: UK Commission for Employment and Skills.

Wintour, P. (2014) More sanctions imposed on jobseeker's allowance claimants, www.theguardian.com/politics/2014/may/14/more-jobseekers-allowance-claimants-subject-benefit-sanctions (accessed 3 December 2014).

Woodruff, W. (2002) *The Road to Nab End: An extraordinary Northern childhood.* London: Abacus.

Worley, C. (2005) 'It's not about race. It's about community': New Labour and community cohesion. *Critical Social Policy* 25, 4, 483–496.

Wymer, W. and Starnes, B. (2001) Conceptual foundations and practical guidelines for recruiting volunteers to serve in local nonprofit organizations: Part 1. *Journal of Nonprofit and Public Sector Marketing* 9, 1, 63–96.

INDEX

ABCD (Achieving Better Community Development) model of evaluation 196–7, 202
accessibility of services 77, 157–9, 184
accomodation *see* housing
accountability 88; circles of 74–5
ADHD (Attention Deficit Hyperactivity Disorder) 65, 76, 80, 97
adolescence: anti-social behaviour 89, 93, 96; individualisation 88; mental health 51, 61; relationships 91; sexual exploitation 100; single parenthood 32; and social work values 38 *see also* young people
adult social care 110–31; case studies 116, 123–4, 129–30; disability/ill health 120–5; and exclusion 110–16; older people 125–30; outcomes framework 113–14; participation 55; personalisation and independence 116–20
adulthood: transition into 87–8, 103–4, 164
advising claimants 45–6
advocacy: adult social care 113–14, 118, 121, 123–4, 126; and the benefits system 48–9; disability 7, 123–4; evaluation 195; older people 126; parents as advocates 102–3; racism and asylum seekers 182, 184; self-advocacy 58; social work values 26, 28–9, 33, 37–8; tackling exclusion in practice 43, 47–9, 52, 55, 58
Age UK 19, 125, 127, 129, 141
ageing populations 158
ageism 125
agency 20, 87–8, 129, 135
Alinsky, S. 144–5
Allen, D. 183, 185
Allen, G. 75
ambiguities of social exclusion 8–9
ambivalence towards poverty 25–6
annual monitoring of social exclusion 8–9
anti-oppressive practice 25
anti-racist practice 172, 174

anti-social behaviour 78–9; young people 93–6
Applebee, E. 191
Arnstein's Ladder 56
assessment: children in need 67–70, 101; disability 46, 83; formal 25–6; self-assessment 119; work capability 48, 122–4
associational networks 175
asylum seekers 11, 176–83; advocacy 182, 184; children as 179, 181–2; community links 183; destitution among 178–9; education 183; gender issues 177, 179–81; housing 179–81, 183; promoting inclusion 182–3; sexual exploitation 180; women as 179–81
Atos 123
austerity 1–2, 8, 28, 36, 130
Axford, N. 20, 68, 76

Baby Safe 162
Backwith, D. 27
Baldwin, N. 64, 66, 70
Ball, S. 108
Barnardo's 97, 105–6
Barnardo's Works project 92
Barnes, J. 85, 147
Barr, A. 112, 160, 196–8
Bateman, N. 49
bedroom tax 33–4
behaviour: anti-social 20, 64–5, 67, 75, 78, 88–9, 93–6, 184, 192–3; children's 51, 64–5, 68, 70, 75, 78, 80–1, 88–90; gateway 70; and gender 88–90, 97; group-level 60; individual 20, 25, 81; need to change/control 29, 31–2, 38–9, 43, 51, 53, 60, 69, 78, 129, 201; parenting 68, 184; protective 73; and racism 170–1, 174–5, 184; sexual 90–1, 100–2
benefits 30, 36, 49, 163; Child Tax Credit 47, 178; council tax support 33–4; eligibility criteria 4, 7, 19, 29, 33, 43–7, 82, 114,

on social work values 31–6; risk shift 29; sanctions system 29–31
welfare state 1, 5, 16, 25, 28–9, 31, 36–7, 148
Wilkinson, D. 191
women asylum seekers 179–81
work *see* employment
work capability assessment 48, 122–4
Work Programmes 48, 125
Working Tax Credit 33, 47; Child Tax Credit 47, 178; family tax credits 63; working families tax credits 8
Working Together 70
worklessness 31, 37, 63
work-readiness 16

YiPPEE (Young People in Care - Pathways to Education in Europe) study 102
young people 86–109; anti-social behaviour 93–6; austerity 36; and benefit sanctions 45; building relationships 91–3; care leavers 102–8; case studies 95–6, 101–2, 106–7; exclusion 86–91; leaving care 103–4; reparative relationships with 91–2; rural areas 164–5; safeguarding 98–102; sexual exploitation 97–102
youth offending teams 100
youth services cuts 87, 165